The NEW face of the NHS

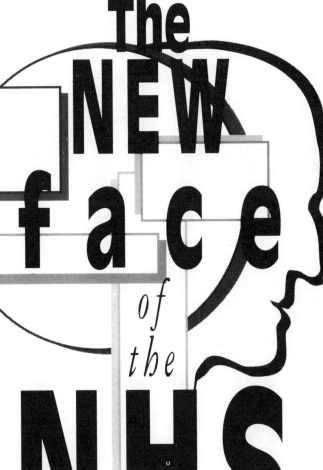

Edited by

Peter Spurgeon

CHURCHILL
LIVINGSTONE

EDINBURGH LONDON MADRID MELBOURNE NEW YORK AND TOKYO 1996

CHURCHILL LIVINGSTONE
Medical Division of Pearson Professional Ltd

British Library Cataloguing in Publication Data
A catalogue record for this book is available from the British Library

First edition 1993
  Reprinted 1996

ISBN 0-582-21998-1

© Longman Group UK Limited 1993
© Pearson Professional Limited 1996

set in 10/11 Garamond
by The Midlands Book Typesetting Co.
Printed in Great Britain by Redwood Books, Trowbridge, Wiltshire

Contents

Foreword

Stuart Dickens

The most significant feature of the post-Griffiths NHS is that Health Authorities will become organisationally and culturally pluralistic.
Professor Derek Williams

When the first edition of this book was written in 1990 no particular prescience was required to anticipate an emerging pluralism and the build up of a major change agenda. However there were few that predicted the extraordinary pace of change or indeed the extent to which the impact of internal market pressures would be evident within 18 months of the introduction of the Government's NHS reforms.

We are seven years on from the introduction of general management and furthermore only a decade from the 1982 reforms which refocussed operational management. The inexorable metamorphosis of NHS management units to Trust status is no more than a powerful reaffirmation of the Government's continuing search for an effective vehicle for locally based service management and a shortening of the administrative tail. The emphasis, albeit belatedly, on the commissioning role of the DHA is the means through which the concern for effectiveness as well as efficiency can now be expressed.

The new role of DHAs with the emphasis on commissioning change offers the first effective mechanism for defining the local health agenda and the distribution of resources against health as well as health care priorities. It is early days but the emphasis on strong purchasing propounded at national and regional levels is not just an antidote to provider dominance – which it is – but an obvious message about defining and implementing the new health agenda clearly delineated in the Government's White Paper *The Health of the Nation*.

Griffiths was strong on the management of change through the general manager; a process geared to a personal vision vested in a newly identified leadership. Sir Roy Griffiths recognised the need for the keepers of the flame who would sustain the spirit of change in the face of a sceptical and even hostile workforce. The champions for the

internal market are less easily discerned and the need for an 'owned'
vision of the future NHS is crucial.

It is still very evident that these profound reforms are not well
understood by the communities we serve nor do they enjoy overt
public support. We need to be mindful of this important cultural
dimension – no one under 50 will have lived within any other
environment than the current health system. Mark G Field in his
introduction to a study of comparative health services (1989)[1] makes
the point that health services around the world 'increasingly share
common elements' but 'it is the particularism of different cultures that
continues to produce that variety and diversity we see in health systems
around the world'. He goes on to emphasise that this feature of health
systems 'puts some limit on the degree to which organisational features
and even medical technology can be transferred from one society to
another'. The vocabulary of the health market is not the natural language
within our national culture and this dissonance compounds public and
to some extent professional anxieties. However notwithstanding these
natural concerns about change and discontinuity the present climate is
exhilarating academically and managerially.

The most profound change is the newly defined role of the District
Health Authority. The notion that Health Authorities should be
concerned with health status and the reduction of morbidity and
mortality is not new, but the preventative dimension of the 1946
Act was lost in the pressing business of running hospitals and
treating, as far as resources would allow, the presenting workload.
That Health Authorities, as their prime responsibility, should make
the essential relationship between need and available resources is a
major step forward. We will now see Health Authorities making overt
decisions about the differential priorities between health and health
care programmes rather than the trade off between inputs (wards, staff
and physical resources) that is the conventional response to financial
pressure in a cash limited system.

The membership of District Health Authorities has been subject to
considerable analysis and comment. Anxieties about male middle class
dominance have to be taken seriously if the Health Authority is to be
seen as the authoritative voice for health in its community.

If the separation of purchaser and provider is to secure benefits for
the health strategist as well as those concerned with service delivery,
we need to critically examine the current membership of DHAs
which were set up when direct management remained a pressing
imperative. It is important for the NHS to become more businesslike as
Kenneth Clarke emphasised, however, the businessman's contribution
may be less relevant in the world of health needs assessment, health
gain and the less easily defined DHA/community interface.

The next three years, and more likely five, will be a period of
transition. We are already experiencing the disorientation that comes
from rapid change and a stumbling articulation of a number of key
issues and their consequences. We must create a learning environment

and see the development of a number of these innovations in an action learning context. Whatever imperatives are built into plans and timetables, the process of lasting change and 'owned' outcomes must transcend deadlines and due dates. Changes will be behavioural as well as structural. Structure is less important than the way our health care organisations behave. Quality depends crucially on a value driven management not structural change. The notion that the patient, client or carer should influence the shape and style of service provision challenges providers and purchasers alike. In Birmingham the Community Care Special Action Project gave a platform to the voice of consumers and carers. The messages are uncomfortable and often at odds with the 'professional' view of the customers' needs and the service response. At the end of the project they are still learning how to insinuate the consumers' perspective into both service delivery and service development.

As these chapters were being finalised the implementation of the government community care reforms were well advanced. Much of the anxiety about the brittleness of historic relationships between the NHS and Local Authorities has been overcome as both face up to the force majeure of the transfer of responsibility to Local Authorities for placing people in residential and nursing home care as well as implementing individual programmes for domiciliary support. However these important reforms are being implemented amidst a backdrop of a dramatically changing public service environment which reinforces Charles Handy's observations about the role of managers 'finding pathways through discontinuous change'. Again the imperatives of reform are creating real and hopefully lasting alliances.

There remains of course a continuing angst about structure: the scale of purchasing authorities; Trust configurations; the cost benefits of large as opposed to small organisations; the danger of monopoly providers (and more recently monopoly purchasers). Historically the NHS has always anguished about size and structure but in truth if we listen to the current newspeak – practice sensitive purchasing; locality based purchasing; 'local voices'; commissioning, purchasing and contracting; preferred providers and contestability; market entrance and exit strategies; market pressures and market management – we hear the vocabulary of a new and developing environment. A shorthand which defines major behavioural as well as process changes about which we know little and are now beginning to learn a great deal. Some aspects of the change agenda will inevitably be handled less well than others. We will need to accept that a mature management recognises the lessons of failure and learns from the experience of doing.

Increasingly close collaboration between academics and service professionals, commissioners and providers, is essential if we are going to focus the change agenda, and more importantly, understand the new dynamic. The new roles of DHAs, Trusts and GP fund holders are shaping that new dynamic which in turn will demand new skills and a rethink of the way health institutions work. The internal health market clearly challenges most of the conventions that have been a feature of NHS culture since its inception, and whilst much of current activity is driven by the imperative to determine how the new order will work most of the required change is crucially dependent on individual and organisational behaviour. Failure to recognise this will create dysfunction and disappointment.

This book makes an important contribution to the learning environment. Rosebeth Moss Kanter (1990)[2] emphasises that 'a learning attitude is a clear necessity in new ventures but it is also needed for achieving synergies and for discovering the benefits of strategic alliances'. These synergies and alliances are evident in the chapters that follow. That we shall not meet all our targets and that some of the systems will prove less than effective vehicles for delivering policy objectives should not surprise us. The opportunities and challenges should shape the learning agenda, and we in turn should learn to be comfortable with a less than seamless robe at least in the short term.

References

Field, Mark G (ed) (1989) *Success and Crisis in National Health Systems* Routledge, p. 21.
Kanter, RM (1990) *When Giants Learn to Dance* Simon and Schuster.

Contributors

Stuart Dickens	Senior Consultant, Dearden Management
Peter Spurgeon	Director of Research and Consultancy, Health Services Management Centre
Chris Ham	Director, Health Services Management Centre
Penelope Mullen	Lecturer, Health Services Management Centre
Tony Cook	Head of Finance Studies, Health Services Management Centre
Mike Drummond	Professor of Economics, University of York
David Thompson	Lecturer, Health Services Management Centre
Hugh Flanagan	Associate, Health Services Management Centre
Hugh Koch	Managing Director, Koch Consultancy
David Schofield	Lecturer, Development Administration Group, University of Birmingham
Peter Hatcher	Senior Fellow, Health Services Management Centre
Andrew Willis	Liaison GP, Northampton Health Authority
Michael Tremblay	Lecturer, Health Services Management Centre
Anne Davis	Associate, Health Services Management Centre
Bernard Crump	Consultant in Public Health Medicine, Central Birimingham Health Authority
Rod Griffiths	Professor of Public Health, University of Birmingham
John Dennis	Chief Executive, Richmond, Twickenham and Roehampton NHS Trust

1 The development of the purchasing function

Chris Ham and Peter Spurgeon

The emergence of purchasing

In the period after publication of *Working for Patients*, (Department of Health 1989) attention focused mainly on the two major innovations contained in the White Paper: NHS trusts and GP fund holding. There was much less debate about the new role of Health Authorities as purchasers of services on behalf of local people. With the passage of time, this has begun to change, and there is now widespread agreement that the development of the purchasing function is crucial to the successful implementation of the NHS reforms. The decision of the Secretary of State to earmark £10m nationally to develop the role of Health Authorities, announced in February 1992, sent out a clear signal of the importance that the Government attaches to purchasing.

Underpinning this shift of emphasis was increasing recognition throughout the NHS that purchasing did not simply involve minor adjustments to the role of Health Authorities but rather required a fundamental change of approach. As experience gained in implementing the reforms showed, Health Authorities had to be more than just contracting agencies responsible for negotiating the providers and monitoring the operations of contracts in practice. Purchasing involved a much wider range of responsibilities including assessing the population's need for health care, evaluating the effectiveness of services, engaging in a dialogue with GPs, involving the public, working in collaboration with other agencies and determining priorities for the use of scarce resources. Discharging these responsibilities effectively called for the creation of organisations capable of breaking away from a tradition of provider dominance in the NHS and taking on the role of champions of the people. These lessons from experience of making the reforms work at a local level were publicised in a series of reports from Project 26 in the Department of Health and from other sources (see for example Department of Health 1990, 1991, and Ham 1990a, Ham and Heginbotham 1991) and they helped to ensure that purchasing moved up the policy and management agenda.

Purchasing in practice

Creating purchasing organisations

At an early stage, it was recognised that the development of the purchasing function would entail a reduction in the number of Health Authorities. This was never stated explicitly in Department of Health guidance but those charged with responsibility for implementing the NHS reforms saw mergers as a natural consequence of the establishment of NHS trusts and the parallel development of a strategic purchasing capacity. In many places, the emphasis was placed on joint working between Health Authorities, often through purchasing consortia, as the first step on the road to mergers. A review of the development of joint purchasing in six areas identified a number of reasons behind the initiatives that had been taken and these are summarised in Box 1.1.

Box 1.1 Reasons for joint purchasing

Some DHAs too small to form viable purchasing organisations

Shortage of people with skills in purchasing

Achieves economies of scale

Greater financial leverage will be available

Increases the potential of competition among providers

Makes it easier to form healthy alliances with FHSAs and Local Authorities

Assists in the integrated purchasing and provision of primary care, community care and secondary care

Source: Ham and Heginbotham 1991

Alongside organisational change at the Health Authority level, increasing effort was put into thinking through the management arrangements needed within Health Authorities to support purchasing. Compared with the old style authorities, it was recognised that purchasing organisations needed fewer staff but that these staff would often be senior personnel with extensive managerial experience. Depending on the size of the authority, headquarters organisations ranging from around 30 to 60 were envisaged, the main functions involved being public health, finance and planning or contracting. In addition, many purchasers sought to acquire expertise in the fields of quality management, public relations, health economics and information technology.

In view of the size of purchasing organisations, and the wide range of tasks to be undertaken, a considerable emphasis was placed on the need for flexible methods of working. Establishing strong individual departments – in finance, public health and other functions – was seen as less important than encouraging corporate working in multidisciplinary teams. Again, no single model emerged, but the principle of flexible functioning was widely seen as a desirable aim, even if most authorities fell short of this in practice.

In the light of growing awareness of the magnitude of the changes facing Health Authorities, increasing importance was attached to developing organisations able to take on purchasing work. This involved investing time and resources in the development of individual managers and Health Authorities and corporate bodies. Central to this process was the establishment of a shared vision of the purpose of purchasing and the objectives it was intended to achieve at a local level. In many cases, the vision included a commitment to creating outward looking organisations embedded in local communities and working with other agencies to improve the population's health. Setting aside time to clarify the vision behind purchasing and ensuring that the vision was widely shared and communicated was a key element in changing the culture of Authorities and developing a corporate approach to purchasing. Much less attention was paid to the equally important issue of how purchasing decisions would be implemented, particularly when they involve significant changes in resource allocation.

Forging purchaser alliances

One of the first lessons learnt by Health Authorities in taking on their new purchasing responsibilities was the importance of working in collaboration with other agencies and interests. This applied particularly to GPs who occupied a pivotal position between purchasers, providers and patients. With GPs responsible for referring patients to hospital for diagnosis and treatment, and Health Authorities responsible for placing contracts with hospitals, there was an obvious requirement that Health Authorities and GPs should work together to decide what services should be purchased and where contracts should be placed.

In recognition of this, Health Authorities used a variety of methods to consult GPs and seek their views. These methods included questionnaire surveys, visits to individual practices and meetings at which GPs were invited to state their opinions on services and identify areas for improvement. In some Authorities, GPs were appointed as members of the purchasing teams established by Health Authorities and participated in advisory committees set up to provide feedback on the new contracting arrangements.

The messages coming back from GPs helped Health Authorities to determine priorities. This included not only tackling long standing problems like waiting times for treatment, it also meant responding to the concern of GPs to have better access to services like physiotherapy and chiropody. The significance of this was that physiotherapy and chiropody were not high priorities in the past because priorities were shaped by the demands of hospital doctors. As GPs were more closely involved in advising Health Authorities, priorities started to change and resources were allocated in different ways. To begin with the effect was felt mainly at the margins but the dialogue between Health Authorities and GPs indicated the shape of things to come.

The involvement of GPs in purchasing was reinforced by closer collaboration between Health Authorities and FHSAs. Over a period of years, FHSAs have shifted from being 'pay and rations' bodies responsible for administering the contracts of family practitioners into planning agencies with greater powers to shape the pattern of services in their areas. This was illustrated by the allocation of a cash limited budget to FHSAs for the improvement of practice premises and the employment of practice staff. The use of this budget enabled FHSAs to target resources where they were most needed, thereby raising standards of primary care.

As a consequence of this and other changes, FHSAs and DHAs have moved closer together, at least in terms of the functions they perform. Both are concerned with assessing health care needs and allocating resources in response to these needs. Furthermore, the two kinds of authority have been enjoined to work with each other to help achieve the objectives set out in *The Health of the Nation* and to ensure seamlessness in the delivery of services. The importance of joint working is exemplified in relation to community nursing where there is plenty of scope for duplication in service provision and competition for scarce staff unless DHAs and FHSAs are acting in concert.

Beyond these considerations, the increasing interest shown by many DHAs in consulting with GPs on the development of their plans indicated that DHAs were beginning to think outside their traditional concerns with acute hospital services. Indeed, some Authorities were further to facilitate work by GPs and consultants to develop protocols for the treatment of common conditions such as asthma and diabetes. One of the purposes of these protocols was to encourage GPs to take on an enhanced role in the provision of services and to reduce the inappropriate use of specialist care. In addition, a few Authorities allocated resources directly to GPs to enable them to assume additional responsibilities. To support developments such as these, DHAs and FHSAs established a variety of initiatives designed to promote joint working (see Box 1.2). These initiatives encompassed the appointment of a chief executive to serve both authorities, the establishment of a shared executive team, the creation of a single budget for community services and general medical services under the joint control of the FHSA and DHA, and the appointment of an FHSA chief executive to manage both family health services and the DHA's community services.

Box 1.2 Collaboration between DHAs and FHSAs: some examples

Doncaster, Gwent and Dorset appointed a single Chief Executive to serve both types of authority

Barking, Havering and Brentwood undertook joint needs assessment for particular localities and client groups and created a single budget for some services under the joint control of the two Authorities

In Stockport the DHA and FHSA were known as the Stockport NHS Authorities and established close collaboration at all levels

Wolverhampton appointed the DHA Chief Executive as Chief Executive (Purchasing) for the FHSA and the FHSA Chief Executive took on the role of General Manager for a combined community services and primary care unit

Wessex RHA has established Health Commissions with enlarged geographic boundaries based on a virtual merger of DHA and FHSA

More generally, there was increasing interest in joint appointments in relation to public health and contracting, and in the production of joint reports and surveys. As time went on, FHSAs also played an increasingly active part in purchasing consortium arrangements, in some regions taking the leading role in these arrangements (eg North East Thames). The extent of collaboration across the country should not be exaggerated, and in some places little progress was made, but overall the impression that emerged was of joint working serving as the forerunner to the eventual merger of DHAs and FHSAs.

Initially, DHAs paid less attention to Local Authorities than to GPs and FHSAs. This was understandable in a period when the agenda was fully taken up with implementing the NHS reforms but it became less tenable as the 1993 deadline for implementing the community care reforms approached. In this respect, the preparation of community care plans gave greater salience to the role of Local Authorities and highlighted the need for purchasing activity to encompass Social Service Authorities as well as NHS Authorities. Guidance issued by the Department of Health underlined the importance of collaboration and outlined the key tasks that needed to be undertaken to ensure the effective implementation of the community care reforms.

The other key dimension of purchaser alliances concerned relationships with providers. As an increasing number of directly managed units became NHS trusts, Health Authorities had to learn to work with providers on a more equal basis than had often been the case in the past. To begin with, this caused difficulties on both sides. In particular, some purchasers and providers tended to adopt an aggressive attitude towards each other, not recognising the need to work in collaboration to achieve benefits for patients.

Put another way, Health Authorities and NHS Trusts struggled to establish effective contracting relationships in place of line management relationships. Consequently, unrealistic stances were taken in negotiations over contracts, with purchasers demanding standards that could not be achieved and providers requiring resources that were not available. To a large extent these were teething problems born out of lack of familiarity with operating under changed circumstances but they illustrated the distance that had to be travelled before a new equilibrium could be struck. There is developing a more realistic and mature relationship between purchasers and providers such that collaborative, longer term contracts are being considered and both parties are able to work cooperating to maximise the effective use of resources. This is particularly valuable in terms of managing clinical innovation and also where radical change in service provisions is suggested.

Involving the public

A specific example of purchaser alliances, deserving treatment in its own right, concerns public participation in the purchasing process. The reason for singling this out for special consideration is that the NHS reforms offer an opportunity to transform Health Authorities from provider dominated organisations into agencies acting as champions of the people. It is this notion that has caught the imagination of ministers and that has stimulated Health Authorities to explore various mechanisms for involving the public in their decisions.

An early review of the experiences of six DHAs identified a number of initiatives that had been taken (see Box 1.3), and a more recent study has described in detail the wide range of approaches that have been pursued (Department of Health 1992a). These approaches include developing explicit strategies for communicating with the public, ensuring that local voices are heard through CHCs, public meetings, and voluntary groups, carrying out surveys of public opinion, and building in a locality focus to purchasing. While much of this work is not new, going back at least to the 1960s when public participation first came into vogue, the separation of purchaser and provider roles in the NHS gives it added significance by enabling Health Authorities to think afresh about the way in which they arrive at their decisions and the part to be played by the public in this process.

These issues are particularly important in view of the new composition of Health Authorities. Compared with the old style NHS, DHAs contain fewer members drawn from local communities and managers occupy up to one half of the places that are available. As a consequence, Health Authorities have to find other ways of demonstrating that they are genuinely acting on behalf of local people. It is this that helps to explain the widespread interest in involving the public in purchasing.

Box 1.3 Involving the public: early initiatives

Giving priority to public relations

Commissioning market research

Carrying out surveys of patients' views

Organising meetings with local voluntary organisations

Arranging public meetings to explain the DHA's new role and responsibilities

Undertaking life style surveys of local residents

Working closely with the CHC

Source: Ham and Matthews 1991

In addition, there is increasing recognition that the purpose of Health Authorities should be to distance themselves from providers and use their purchasing power to negotiate improvements in services for the people they serve. This is the *raison d'etre* of Health Authorities under the NHS reforms and one of the yardsticks against which their performance will be judged. The logic here is that by breaking the umbilical cord which in the past has tied providers to Health Authorities, the reforms create an opportunity for resources to be used in a way which better meets the population's needs. It is this idea which lies behind the vision that many purchasers have developed to guide their activities and which offers the potential for giving the public a bigger say in what services should be provided and where.

Against this background, a number of Authorities have shown particular interest in locality purchasing. In large part, this has been prompted by the move to merge Health Authorities and create purchasing consortia. In many parts of the NHS, a serious attempt is being made to balance the advantages of joint purchasing with initiatives designed to ensure that purchasers remain sensitive to the needs of small areas. To this end, Authorities are exploring ways in which they can build a locality focus into their work.

Assessing needs

Information obtained from local people provides Health Authorities with a source of intelligence about the needs they are expected to meet. This information is often characterised as 'soft' data and can be contrasted with hard data about patterns of illness and mortality in each district. Hard data usually defines needs in quantitative terms making use of available statistics on the health of the population. Soft data is more often presented in terms of the views and opinions of local people, and as such may reflect demands rather than needs. However, local views are sometimes assessed on a systematic basis through survey research and when this happens soft data may be presented in a quantified fashion.

All Health Authorities rely to an increasing extent on the annual reports prepared by their Directors of Public Health for information about health care needs. These reports have become more sophisticated over time and in most districts now provide a sound basis on which to make purchasing decisions. As well as painting a picture of health in each district, public health reports seek to look at the balance of expenditure on different services and the relative cost effectiveness of this expenditure. This is central to the purchasing function in that it enables Health Authorities to raise questions about the appropriateness of historical spending patterns and to explore options for reallocating resources into alternative areas of service provision.

In this context, the Department of Health has sought to support the work of Health Authorities by developing a number of central initiatives. These include funding a needs network at the Institute of Public Health at Birmingham University, supporting the preparation of a series of effectiveness bulletins by the Universities of Leeds and York, and initiating work on health care outcomes. In addition, the Department has commissioned a programme of research reviews on selected health care topics. The reviews go under the title of epidemiologically based needs assessments and initially covered diabetes, hip and knee joint replacement, stroke and renal disease. In these ways, the Department was able to avoid Health Authorities re-inventing the wheel, and it encouraged the spread of good practices throughout the NHS.

Reviewing experience of health needs assessment, the DHA project in the Department of Health identified three approaches (Department of Health 1991). These were:

- Epidemiological assessments based on the ability to benefit from health care and reflecting evidence on incidence, prevalence and cost effectiveness of treatments;

- Comparative assessments reviewing the local use of services and the performance of providers against what is achieved elsewhere; and

- A corporate approach which takes account of the various interests of the different groups involved including local people, GPs, other agencies, providers, regions and the Management Executive.

In reality, purchasers found that they had to use all three approaches, balancing the harder data coming out of epidemiological and comparative assessments with the softer data involved in the corporate approach. However, there remains a problem of translating information from the public into explicit purchasing decisions.

Making choices

The purpose of assessing needs is not to prepare an ever more detailed profile of the population's health as an end in itself. Rather, it is to help Health Authorities decide what services they wish to purchase with the resources at their disposal. As many observers have noted, the separation of purchaser and provider roles makes decision making more explicit than in the past. This is because Health Authorities have to set out in contracts those services they wish to purchase. The corollary is that contracts will reveal which services are not purchased, either because resources are not available or because purchasers deem these services to be low priority.

The question this raises is how should purchasers reach decisions on priorities? In an ideal world, it would be possible to assemble information about the costs and effectiveness of different services and rank them in order of priority. In practice, information on costs and effectiveness is seriously incomplete. In any case, priority setting still requires those charged with making decisions to exercise their judgement on the use of resources. (Heginbotham, Ham *et al.*, 1992).

In the past, priority setting in the NHS has been inherently a political process. The policies and priorities established by health ministers have been communicated to Health Authorities who have interpreted national policies to suit local circumstances. As part of this process, Health Authorities have been influenced strongly by professional views, particularly those emanating from doctors working in the acute hospital sector. It is in this sense that Health Authorities have often been captured by providers who have been able to win a bigger share of resources for their services.

The NHS reforms challenge this approach to policy making in a number of ways. First, by separating purchaser and provider roles, the reforms may enable Health Authorities to take a view on priorities that is more independent of provider interests. There is already evidence that this is happening as Health Authorities, in conjunction with GPs, seek to hold hospital providers more accountable for their performance.

Second, the reforms also offer an opportunity for purchasing decisions to reflect more accurately the views of local people. As noted above, in their new purchasing role, Health Authorities have taken a variety of initiatives to involve the public in decision making, in an attempt to gain credibility and legitimacy for their role as champions of the people. In the longer term, these initiatives may enable Health Authorities to draw systematically on public preferences in shaping their priorities.

A third implication of the reforms is that purchasers should examine the cost effectiveness of the services available. This has been identified as a central feature of the purchasing function in guidance issued by

Figure 1.1

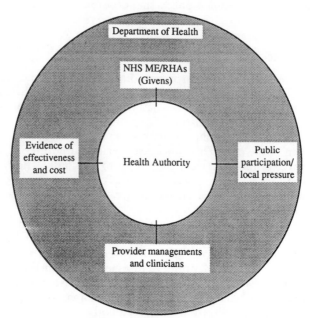

Source: Heginbotham, Ham et. al. 1992

the Department of Health. As the guidance has emphasised, purchasers need to ensure that they obtain good value for money by concentrating their expenditure on those services which offer the greatest benefit at least cost. To help Health Authorities in this task, the Department has commissioned a series of studies to make available the results of evaluation research to Health Authorities.

The effect of these changes is illustrated in Figure 1.1. The figure was developed in a simulation of the priority setting process undertaken jointly by the Southampton and West Hampshire Health Authority and the King's Fund College. During the simulation, it was argued that in the past decisions in DHAs were strongly influenced by national and regional priorities on the one hand, and the views of local professionals on the other. To this extent, the vertical axis has been to the fore.

The NHS reforms offer the opportunity of placing greater emphasis on the horizontal axis, in the form of the views of local people and evidence drawn from cost effectiveness studies. This is not to suggest that decision making will cease to be a political process. Rather, it is to argue that one of the aims of the reforms is to alter the basis on which decisions are formulated and to change the balance of power between different interests. Judgements and values will continue to be important, as will lobbying and other forms of political activity, but the aspiration at least is to give more attention to elements which in the past have not received as much priority.

This conclusion is consistent with experience in the State of Oregon of setting priorities within the Medicaid programme (see Box 1.4). As those charged with priority setting in Oregon discovered, the process of ranking different services cannot be reduced to a technical exercise in which decisions are reached on the basis of evidence alone. In reality, evidence has to be weighed in the context of community values as well as in relation to the public's perception of priorities. In this respect, the process of priority setting may be just as important as the outcome.

Box 1.4 The Oregon approach

The State of Oregon developed its work on rationing and priority setting as a result of difficulties in funding the Medicaid programme. The Oregon approach has evolved over time but essentially it involves an attempt to define a basic set of services to be provided to people eligible under Medicaid. The method used starts from an analysis of the costs and benefits of the different services. These services are ranked in order of priority to produce a league table of interventions. In parallel, information is gathered on the community's values and preferences through public hearings, town hall meetings and other approaches. Using this information, the commissioners who oversee the process discuss and debate priorities, and make recommendations to the legislature. Ultimately, the availability of resources determines what services are included in the Oregon Medicaid scheme but what characterises the Oregon approach is the attempt to combine technical information drawn from scientific studies with intelligence about community values.

Put slightly differently, if it is accepted that making choices on the use of scarce resources does not admit of a single right answer, then it follows that the method used to arrive at these choices should be open and amenable to the influence of different interests. This will enable different options to be tested rigorously and it will allow the strengths and weaknesses of alternative investment strategies to be assessed. Research results should contribute to decision making wherever they are available but so too should soft data about community values and opinions. Ultimately, decision makers (whether state commissioners in Oregon or DHAs in the UK) have to arrive at their own judgements on priorities, but if the process of setting priorities is robust this will make it easier to defend and justify the decisions that are made. It may also result in better decisions.

Developing contracts

Discussion of the role of contracts in purchasing has deliberately been placed towards the end of this chapter to put contracts in their proper context. Experience has demonstrated that purchasing is not the same as contracting, involving as it does the range of strategic tasks already discussed. Nevertheless, the outcome of purchaser alliances, involving the public, assessing needs and making choices is the negotiation of contracts with providers for the delivery of services. As the vehicle for implementing purchasing decisions, contracts thus have a vital part to play in the new NHS.

With the exception of GP fund holders, most contracts in 1991/2 were block contracts. These described in broad terms the range of services providers were expected to deliver. Contracts usually specified both the cost and volume of services but often at a general level. As well as specifying cost and volume, contracts included a range of quality standards. For the most part, these standards concerned the environment of care and patient convenience rather than clinical issues. Typical examples of standards included maximum waiting times for appointments and the speed at which discharge information should be communicated to GPs.

Given the general nature of most contracts in the first year, purchasers had few levers at their disposal with which to improve performance. Set against this, they were at least protected against demands for extra resources from providers who exceeded the activity levels contained in contracts. In view of the increases in activity reported across the NHS in 1991/2, this was not unimportant. But ultimately, block contracts with broad cost and volume indicators which were not linked to rewards and penalties, appeared to offer little advance on the NHS before the reforms. In particular, providers who increased activity beyond the level negotiated with purchasers were still faced with an efficiency trap because additional resources did not follow patients. While it could be claimed that contracts did serve to make standards more explicit, thereby providing a framework for holding providers accountable, in reality there was little evidence that this in itself led to significant service improvements.

Indeed as experience demonstrated, there was little point in purchasers specifying standards in detail if they lacked the means to monitor whether these standards were achieved in practice. As a study of the impact of contracts on quality demonstrated, for the most part monitoring systems were underdeveloped, and were in any case undermined by the lack of readily available information on a number of the areas in contracts covered by standards (Ham *et al.*, 1992). Although a variety of monitoring mechanisms were put in place, taken together they fell short of what was required to enable quality fo be monitored on a systematic basis.

A significant lesson followed on from this, namely that contracts were less important as a tool for improving performance than the relationships that were established between purchasers and providers. In this respect, there was increasing recognition that commercial organisations where purchasing and manufacturing were separated offered a model which might be emulated in the NHS. An often quoted example is Marks and Spencer which buys all of its goods and services from outside suppliers.

The relationship between Marks and Spencer and its suppliers is one of inter-dependence in which the success of the purchaser depends on the success of the providers and vice versa. This creates a common interest in working together to meet the demands of customers (Ham 1990b).

One of the features of Marks and Spencer is that it works in partnership with suppliers to develop new products and to improve quality. There is a genuine sharing of ideas and expertise with staff from Marks and Spencer's head office operating alongside suppliers to produce goods according to the required specifications. Factories operate an open door policy and M and S itself pursues a policy of constructive interference to ensure that its standards are achieved.

NHS experience also demonstrated that contracts needed to include more explicit incentives if they were to be effective. In 1991/2, patients on the whole followed the money, rather than money following patients. This meant that there was little incentive for providers to improve their performance, at least in terms of attracting additional resources from purchasers. Indeed, providers often complained that while the sanctions within contracts were evident, for example, involving resources being removed if targets were not achieved, there was little evidence that rewards were available where targets were exceeded. The difficulty for purchasers was that faced with a cash limit budget there were risks involved in developing sophisticated contracts which linked resources directly with activity. It was therefore unclear how a contracting system could be developed which would both avoid the efficiency trap and enable purchasers to keep expenditure within budget.

The other lesson from the first year of contracting was that extra contractual referrals (ECRs) provided valuable information to purchasers about referral patterns and the strengths and weaknesses of the services for which they had placed contracts. Although covering a small proportion of overall expenditure (usually about 2 per cent of budget), and taking up a disproportionate amount of administrative time, ECRs contained pointers to services with which GPs were dissatisfied. ECRs also caused DHAs to raise questions about the appropriateness of certain referrals. This applied particularly to high cost referrals and to those where there was little evidence that treatments would benefit patients (or at least provide additional benefits over and above those offered by services already under contract).

For the most part, it appeared that DHAs sought to accommodate GPs' requests for ECRs, but there was some evidence that authorities were beginning to enter into a debate with GPs about the need for certain referrals. In this sense, the small proportion of overall expenditure allocated to ECRs came in for closer scrutiny than the much bigger volume of spending on block contracts. The reason, of course, was that ECR expenditure was more visible and had to be approved by purchasers. Nevertheless, experience gained in assessing the appropriateness of ECRs indicated how purchasers might review more rigorously the use of the remaining 98 per cent of their budgets.

Shifting to primary care

The NHS reforms are not intended to radically change the organisation of the NHS and leave the existing pattern of spending and service provision untouched. The point of the changes discussed in this paper is to increase efficiency and make services more responsive to users. The reforms are also designed to promote the policy objectives set out in *The Health of the Nation*. The Green Paper more than any other single document crystallises the ends to which purchasing activity is (or should be) directed. Central to the implementation of the national health strategy is a shift in service provision away from secondary care and towards primary care (including prevention).

There is already evidence that this had started to happend (see Box 1.5). As a result of the developing dialogue between Health Authorities and GPs, not only are hospital providers having to adjust their methods of working, but also there is a movement of the site of care in the direction of GPs. In part, this can be seen in the work going into the development of protocols by GPs and consultants for the treatment of conditions such as asthma and diabetes (see above). One of the purposes of such protocols is to give GPs an enhanced role in the delivery of services with appropriate specialist support. As this work is extended more generally through the NHS, it is likely that other GPs will play a bigger part in providing care for their patients.

Box 1.5 The shift to primary care

The purchasing function has already resulted in a shift to primary care. Not only have DHAs started getting closer to GPs, but also the balance of power within the NHS is changing. Hospital providers are beginning to become more accountable for their performance, and the site of service provision is moving towards primary care. Examples include:

- consultants carrying out out-patient clinics in GPs' surgeries;

- consultants and GPs agreeing shared care arrangements in areas such as asthma, diabetes, psychiatry and maternity care;

- GPs carrying out more minor surgery themselves;

- GPs doing more diagnostic tests in their surgeries, thereby reducing demands on hospitals;

- GPs employing additional staff with support from DHAs and FHSAs to enable them to take on extra responsibilities.

Another example relates to minor surgery. The new contract for GPs introduced in 1990 provided financial incentives to encourage GPs to do more work in this area and this has had an effect. The contract has been reinforced by the GP fund holding scheme and also by the interest shown by some DHAs in allocating part of their budget to GPs to do more work themselves.

A third example relates to the change in the balance of power between GPs and hospital consultants. This has forced hospital doctors to pay greater attention to GPs than was often the case in the past and to be more responsible to the demands of GPs. One manifestation of this has been consultants in some districts holding their out-patient clinics in GPs's surgeries rather than in hospitals.

A fourth example concerns the enhanced role of the primary care team. Survey evidence demonstrates that GPs are keen to offer a wider range of services provided they have adequate support. In many cases, this support is now forthcoming, whether through fund holders purchasing the services of physiotherapists and dieticians directly or through Health Authorities giving higher priority to providing these staff to work alongside GPs. Practice nurses are often key people in this process taking on a range of work in association with other members of the primary care team.

To raise these issues is to highlight yet again the key role of GPs in making the reforms work. The point of the examples given above is that the benefits of the reforms have not simply accrued to fund holders. All GPs are now in a position where they can exert more influence over decision making because the separation of purchaser and provider roles has motivated Health Authorities to involve GPs in determining what services should be provided and where. In this sense, DHAs can be likened to purchasing agents acting on behalf of GPs (and their patients) in their negotiations with providers.

It is this idea that lies behind the emergence of practice sensitive purchasing in districts like Bath (see Box 1.6). In essence, practice sensitive purchasing seeks to make Health Authority purchasing decisions sensitive to the needs of GP practices by involving GPs fully in the purchasing process. As such, it offers many of the benefits of the fund holding scheme while containing fewer risks. Not least, from a GP perspective, practice sensitive purchasing enables GPs to have a bigger say over the use of resources without having to take on additional (and often unwanted) management responsibilities.

Despite the attractions of this approach, ministers have indicated that fund holding will be extended to encompass a wider range of practices and additional services. It is therefore likely that an increasing number of GPs will be involved in the fund holding scheme. The question this raises is how will Health Authorities relate to fund holders in the future?

The dilemma here is that Health Authorities and fund holders offer a starkly contrasting approach to purchasing. On the one hand, Health Authorities take a population wide perspective and are concerned to assess needs and purchase services for communities of around 300,000 on average. On the other hand, GP fund holders undertake purchasing from the perspective of the patients on their list and the demands expressed by the patients who present in their surgeries.

Box 1.6 Practice sensitive purchasing

In 1990 the Bath DHA began exploring practice sensitive purchasing. Its aim is to decentralise decision making and to find a way of making DHA purchasing decisions sensitive to the needs and views of GPs. The idea built on work already underway in Bath to survey the views of GPs, talk to GPs in their own surgeries, and to consult with GPs collectively through an advisory council.

In essence, practice sensitive purchasing seeks to establish a notional budget for GPs by allocating the resources available to the DHA on a practice by practice basis. The use that practices make of services will then be monitored and information on the cost of these services fed back to GPs. In this way, practice sensitive purchasing enables the health authority and GPs to examine how resources are used, and it seeks to achieve real GP involvement in purchasing.

Practice sensitive purchasing is being developed with the support of GPs and a feasibility study is currently underway. The idea is seen as an adjunct to GP fund holding, both in seeking to encompass all practices and in covering all services. Fund holders as well as non-fund holders are involved in its development.

While the size of the communities served by Health Authorities is increasing in the wake of mergers, the size of the lists served by fund holders is declining as smaller practices are allowed to participate in the scheme. In simple terms, the choice is between needs-based purchasing for large populations and demand-based purchasing for small populations. And overlaying this dichotomy is the greater sensitivity of fund holders to their patients, based on proximity and familiarity, compared with the greater financial leverage of Health Authorities resulting from the size of the budgets they control.

In reality, the choices may not be as stark as this dichotomy suggests. As already noted, Health Authorities are pursuing a wide range of initiatives to achieve sensitivity to patients and the public, and this is seen as an essential corollary of the move to create fewer, bigger authorities. Equally, there is increasing recognition that GP fund holders should use their resources not only to respond to patient demands but also to meet health care needs.

What this means is as yet unclear, but one scenario is that Health Authorities in the future will negotiate with fund holders to determine local priorities for improving health and health services. This will enable local health goals to be shaped by fund holders, the quid pro quo being that the way in which fund holders use their resources is directed towards the achievement of these goals. The result may be greater constraints on fund holders than at present, but arguably this is essential in a health service where the policies determined by ministers and implemented by Health Authorities still matter.

Not least, if ministers are committed to achieving the strategy set out in *The Health of the Nation*, there has to be a way of linking fund holders' decisions to the priorities adumbrated in the strategy. The consequence in the medium term could well be the emergence of unified purchasing authorities (merged DHAs and FHSAs) responsible for allocating resources to GPs, negotiating with fund holders on the use of these resources, involving non-fund holders in purchasing through surveys, face to face meetings and a locality focus, and purchasing some services (those not included in the fund holding scheme) on behalf of all GPs. This would enable the benefits of the two approaches to purchasing to be combined and would help to ensure that a properly managed market emerged. Whether such an orderly outcome is possible remains uncertain, but something along these lines is needed if the full benefits of purchasing are to be realised in practice.

It follows that there will continue to be a role for Health Authorities in the future, albeit a changed role. The volume of resources Health Authorities control may decline as the number of fund holders increase, but there will always be a need for a local agency capable of assessing health needs and planning the overall pattern of services.

Getting from here to there

The main purpose of this chapter has been to analyse the lessons learned about purchasing in the implementation of the NHS reforms. Implicit in these lessons are a number of pointers to the future. Speculation about future developments is a hazardous enterprise but in drawing the chapter to a close it may be helpful to spell out as clearly as possible the areas in which further development work is needed.

Forging purchaser alliances

Although an encouraging start has been made in involving GPs in purchasing, much remains to be done to ensure effective participation by *all* GPs in the decisions of health authorities. This will require continuing investment in surveys of GPs, face to face interviews, and participation by representatives of GPs in advisory committees and purchasing teams. The importance of this activity is difficult to overestimate and demands on-going effort on the part of purchasers.

Much the same applies to alliances with FHSAs. The current position varies considerably across the country and depends as much of differences in personality and style as on values and philosophies. The

re-alignment of Health Authority boundaries to bring them into line
with those of FHSAs will help to facilitate collaboration but will not
in itself guarantee effective joint purchasing. Experience indicates that
a variety of initiatives are worth pursuing including joint appointments,
the pooling of resources to enable some services to be purchased jointly,
a common approach to needs assessment and to information systems,
and an investment in understanding the role and responsibilities of the
other agencies. RHAs have a part to play in facilitating collaboration
through mechanisms such as joint review meetings and corporate
contracts which encompass both kinds of authority.

Collaboration with local authorities will assume greater prominence
as implementation of the community care reforms gathers pace. The
issues involved in this area are both old and new. They are old in that
much of the work that has gone into joint planning in the last 16 years
remains relevant. The issues are new to the extent that government
policies have placed even greater responsibilities on local authorities
to plan community care.

Arguably, the challenges involved in developing joint purchasing
between Health Authorities and Social Services Authorities are greater
even than the outstanding agenda represented by the implementation of
the NHS reforms. If they are not tackled systematically, there is a risk
that clients and patients will fall between different agencies, and that
seamlessness in service delivery will remain but an empty slogan. And
if, as many of those involved fear, the resources available are inadequate
for the purpose, Health Authorities and Social Services Authorities may
adopt increasingly narrow definitions of their responsibilities, leaving a
grey area in the middle which neither agency will take on.

Establishing a new equilibrium between purchasers and providers
is to a large extent dependent on there being sufficient time for line
management relationships to be replaced by contracting relationships.
The difficulties that have emerged in the first year are a reflection of
the immaturity of the purchaser/provider interface and a demonstration
of the work which still remains to be done. Apart from learning
from experience, Health Authorities and NHS trusts may be able to
shorten the learning curve by studying the experience of successful
commercial organisations like Marks and Spencer (see above). If
nothing else, an analysis of how purchasers and providers (or buyers
and manufacturers) operate outside the health sector will contain
some clues as to traps to be avoided as well as successes to be
emulated.

Involving the public

As champions of the people, Health Authorities have a major job to
do to gain credibility in their new role. It is clear that there is no
one approach that will a achieve this credibility. Purchasers need to
use a variety of mechanisms along the lines that have already been
initiated. Of particular importance is the establishment of a locality

focus to compensate for the remoteness and distance that is inevitably involved in the creation of fewer, bigger authorities. In this respect, the emerging experiments in locality purchasing need to be carefully monitored to establish the lessons for the future.

Also important is the contribution of CHCs who often see themselves as champions of the people. The separation of purchaser and provider roles enables the relationship between Health Authorities and CHCs to be reviewed to explore areas in which CHCs can act in collaboration with Health Authorities. As an example, CHCs could play an important part in helping Health Authorities to monitor standards in contracts from the perspective of patients and the public, thereby helping to fill the gap that exists in this area.

Assessing needs

Needs assessment is a pluralistic endeavour involving the bringing together of hard and soft data from a variety of sources. These sources include intelligence from local people, epidemiological information about patterns of morbidity and mortality, and national studies of particular procedures and services. The state of the art in this area is developing apace and it is vital to avoid wheels being reinvented in different districts. In this regard, the Department of Health has a key role to perform in funding central initiatives, such as the needs network and cost effectiveness bulletins, to provide support to Health Authorities.

For their part, Health Authorities have to build on the foundations established by the annual reports produced by their directors of public health. At one level, the production of these reports needs to be synchronised with the preparation of purchasing plans. At another level, there is a need to ensure that needs assessment is not an academic exercise but has practical applications and relevance to the work of Health Authorities. At this point in the development of purchasing, focussing on a few areas of service provision in which public health analysis can contribute directly to decision making will enable some early successes to be achieved as a basis for more fundamental work at a later stage.

Making choices

The rationing of scarce resources is an inevitable and unenviable task of purchasers. There is no quick fix in this area and to a large extent the process of decision making is as important as the outcome. Given that priority setting is not amenable to right answers, Health Authorities must be able to defend their decisions by demonstrating that they have consulted effectively with relevant interests and have weighed the available evidence carefully. As rationing decisions become more explicit through the use of contracts, the choices made by purchasers will be even more visible and will therefore have to be justified to local people. This process will be easier if Health Authorities have explained the inevitability of rationing and have shared their dilemmas with the end users of services.

In view of increasing public expectations, the debate about priorities will be uncomfortable for all concerned. But if evidence on the cost effectiveness of services (in the form of QALYs and other techniques) is used alongside views from voluntary organisations and public opinion surveys there will at least be a more informed discussion of priority areas of interest. Already, purchasers are experimenting with different approaches and the lessons of these approaches need to be crystallised and disseminated for wider application.

Developing contracts

As the NHS moves beyond the steady state, contracts will become increasingly sophisticated. There may not be a rapid replacement of block contracts by cost and volume and cost per case contracts, but block contracts will become more detailed and a wider range of rewards and penalties (sticks and carrots) will be introduced. Equally important as contracts themselves will be the monitoring systems that are put in place to assess whether the standards specified by purchasers are being achieved. In this area, there is much room for improvement, a variety of tools being used to determine whether providers are delivering what they have agreed to in contracts.

The contribution of CHCs to monitoring has been mentioned already. Also important are GPs and the public. However, GPs and the public will only be effective guardians of standards if they are aware of the standards included in contracts. At present, they are often ignorant of these standards and this suggests that purchasers should make renewed efforts to publicise the standards negotiated with providers. As an example, this might take the form of a simple summary of standards distributed to all households and GP practices with the name of a purchasing officer who could act as a contact point if standards were not met. In one authority, the role of GPs in monitoring is being formalised through the use of a system in which GPs complete a yellow card if providers fail to fulfil their contracts and this card is sent to the purchaser.

As argued above, alliances with providers have to recognise the interdependence of purchasers and providers of the need to establish collaborative long term relationships. This is not to argue that there should be a cosy arrangement in which both sides settle for a quiet life. Rather, it is to acknowledge that in many districts, purchasers and providers will rely on each other to a large extent and will have to work in tandem to improve services. The implication is that adversarial relationships are less relevant than cooperation over a period of years. The main difference from the past is that the separation of purchaser and provider roles should enable purchasers to hold providers more directly accountable for their performance.

Shift to primary care

It cannot be said often enough that purchasing is only a means to an end. The objective of purchasing is to raise standards of health services and to improve the population's health. The latter objective, the centrepiece of *The Health of the Nation*, is dependent on shifting resources and priorities towards primary care and prevention. This has already started to happen even in the first year of the reforms, and the progress made so far has to be consolidated and extended. Central to this process is closer working between GPs and health authorities and between DHAs and FHSAs.

Also important is the relationship that develops between GP fund holders and Health Authorities. The Government has announced its commitment to the extension of fund holding and as a consequence there is an urgent need to think through the future relationship between fund holders and Health Authorities. Patients and the public are most likely to benefit if fund holders and Health Authorities collaborate rather than compete, both through agreeing on the policy objectives to be pursued and by working together in negotiating and monitoring contracts. The alternative would be increasing fragmentation and an NHS in which demands received greater attention than needs. It is difficult to believe that this is the outcome sought by ministers and it is vital that relationship between fund holders and Health Authorities is clarified as soon as possible.

Market management

The way in which many of the issues discussed in this chapter are resolved depends to a large extent on how the emerging market in the NHS is managed. The Government's aim has never been to allow competition to operate untrammelled. Rather, the objective is to introduce a process of *managed competition* in which the incentives of the market (especially money following patients) are combined with regulation or planning.

What has not been determined is where the balance will be struck between competition and management. Will the emphasis be placed on competition with a minimum amount of management? Or will the market be tightly managed with competition occurring only at the margins? With 1991/2 designated as the year of steady state, these questions have not been resolved, and it remains a matter of doubt as to what will happen as the NHS moves beyond steady state.

Current indications are that the market will throw up problems for ministers sooner rather than later. In particular, a number of hospitals in London have been forced to cut back services because they have not attracted the contracts and resources needed to maintain services at previous levels. In this situation, ministers have to decide whether to allow the market to continue to operate, in which case unsuccessful hospitals will have to reduce their services and ultimately close, or whether to intervene by providing extra resources to allow these hospitals to remain open. Although government spokesmen have stated that they will not hesitate from allowing hospitals to close, the strength of their resolve has yet to be fully tested in practice.

More fundamentally, it remains unclear how Regional Health Authorities (RHAs) will relate to purchasers and providers in future. RHAs are already involved in arbitration when disputes arise over contracts, but the precise nature of their responsibilities in relation to market management have yet to be determined.

What is clear is that there does need to be an agency capable of overseeing the operation of the market on behalf of ministers and in a position to intervene in appropriate circumstances. Such an agency would be responsible not only for resolving disputes between purchasers and providers but also for setting the framework in which competition develops. More specifically, the agency would play a part in determining the size and shape of purchasers and providers, planning for education and research requirements, overseeing the distribution of specialist services, including the availability of expensive high technology, and ensuring that access and equity were not undermined as competition increased. The extent to which the agency would be *laissez-faire* or interventionist in its approach is a political decision and can only be determined when ministers have clarified the way in which the reforms are to proceed.

References

Department of Health (1989) *Working for Patients* CMD 555, HMSO
Department of Health (1990) *Developing Districts* HMSO
Department of Health (1991) *Assessing Health Care Needs* HMSO
Department of Health (1992a) *Local Voices* HMSO
Department of Health (1992b) *Purchasing for Population Health Gain* Mimeo
Ham, CJ (1990a) *Holding on While Letting Go* King's Fund College
Ham, CJ (1990b) Health Authorities and the New Contract Culture Speech to NAHA Conference, January 1990
Ham, CJ and Heginbotham, CJ (1991) *Purchasing Together* King's Fund College
Ham, CJ and Matthews, T (1991) *Purchasing with Authority* King's Fund College
Ham, CJ *et al.* (1992) 'Contract culture' *The Health Service Journal* 7 May 1992
Heginbotham, CJ, Ham, CJ, *et al.* (1992) *Purchasing dilemmas* King's Fund College
Spurgeon P (1993) 'Managing the internal market' in Tilley, I (Ed.) *Managing the Internal Market* Chapmans

2 Planning and internal markets

Penelope Mullen

The White Paper *Working for Patients* (DoH 1989a) stated its objectives as:

- *to give patients, wherever they live in the UK, better health care and greater choice of the services available; and*

- *greater satisfaction and rewards for those working in the NHS who successfully respond to local needs and preferences.*

Among the most fundamental of the proposals designed to meet these objectives were changes in the method of allocating resources to Health Authorities and the separation of the provision of health services from their funding, using what many have termed an 'internal market'. How do these proposals affect health care planning – planning to meet the needs of the population, to secure equity and equality and to maximise health?

Allocation of resources

Working for Patients proposed that Regions, and eventually Districts, would be funded on a weighted per capita basis (with an allowance to the Thames Regions for higher prices in London). The previous 'cross-boundary flow adjustment' would be abolished, leaving Districts to 'pay directly for the services provided for their patients by hospitals in other Districts . . .' (DoH 1989a, para. 4.11).

The allocation of resources has been problematic since the establishment of the NHS. Its inheritance, both in terms of capital stock and medical staff, was very unevenly distributed. Resource distribution during the early years of the NHS was based on previous funding with additions for specific developments, thus perpetuating and even exacerbating the inherited geographical inequalities. The 1962 Hospital Plan (MoH 1962) and the 1971 Formula (DHSS 1970) did attempt to reduce these inequalities at Regional level, but inequalities within Regions exceeded those between Regions (Cooper and Culyer 1970). Prior to 1974, however, planning health care and equalising resources below the Regional level was difficult. This was due largely to the absence in the hospital sector of a geographically-based planning and management tier below the level of the Region. The pre-1974 sub-Regional tier, Hospital Management Committees (HMCs), were responsible for running a hospital or a group of hospitals and rarely had specific responsibilities to ensure that the needs of a defined population were met.

New opportunities for sub-Regional planning came in 1974 with the establishment of Area Health Authorities (AHAs) 'with full planning and operational responsibilities ... responsible for the provision of comprehensive health services ...' to a defined population (DHSS 1972). In 1976 the new NHS Planning System was introduced. At the same time, but quite independently, the report of the Resource Allocation Working Party 'The RAWP Report' (DHSS 1976) made proposals for improving geographical equity both between Regions and within Regions. Regional target allocations were to be based on population, weighted by age, sex and Standardised Mortality Ratios (SMRs) (as a proxy for morbidity), and adjusted for 'cross-boundary flows', using average costs per case by specialty applied to patient flows recorded two or three years earlier, to compensate for treating patients from other Regions. Actual allocations to Regions would be adjusted gradually over several years so that they moved towards the target allocations. The RAWP Report proposed that the '... same principles ... should ... be applied to allocations below Regional level' (DHSS 1976).

The RAWP Report and its implementation have been the centre of considerable discussion, analysis and controversy (see Mays and Bevan 1987) which is outside our scope here. However, the cross-boundary flow adjustment had far-reaching implications for health care planning, in particular for equity and priorities, especially at the sub-Regional level. Whilst over the years there had been a considerable amount of work on costing such flows, a more important question from the point of view of planning was the fact that the home (exporting) authority was compulsorily required to pay for such flows whilst having no control over them (Brazier 1986, 1987, Mullen 1986). It was difficult for an authority to pursue its priorities and plan to meet the needs of its population whilst some of its resources were being used to pay for outward flows not figuring in those priorities. Importing authorities, on the other hand, complained that the cross-boundary flow adjustment did not fully compensate for actual workload since, by using average costs, it did not fully cover the costs of treating high-cost cases. Further, the adjustment was based on historical data and, in any case influenced only target allocations and not actual allocations. In addition, various perverse incentives appeared to be built into the system which were not conducive to good planning (Bevan and Brazier 1987).

Indeed, not long after the RAWP Report was published Mullen (1978) suggested that:

> One partial solution to the problem of accounting for intra-regional cross boundary flows would be to allocate resources to authorities taking no account of the cross-boundary flows and to leave them to take the responsibility of paying for their own residents treated elsewhere . . . there would be far more flexibility for the Area planners to arrange health care for their population.

In view of the problems, many Regions modified or even abandoned the RAWP cross-boundary flow adjustment method for their sub-Regional allocations.

Some concern has been expressed over the actual methodology employed in the *Working for Patients* proposals for the allocation of funding (Mays 1989). However, from the point of view of health care planning, the principle of funding authorities on a weighted capitation basis, with no allowance for cross-boundary flow, is to be welcomed. But do the accompanying proposals for the provision of services hinder or help Health Authorities in fulfilling their planning role?

Funding and the provision of services

Internal markets

As noted above, the *Working for Patients* proposals for securing and providing services involve an 'internal market'. The origin of this term is usually attributed to Enthoven (1985a), who explained his proposals thus:

> Each District would receive a RAWP-based per capita revenue and capital allowance. Each DHA would continue to be responsible to provide and pay for comprehensive care for its own resident population, but not for other people without current compensation. It would be paid for emergency services to outsiders at a standard cost. It would be paid for non-emergency services to outsiders at negotiated prices. It would control referrals to providers outside the District and it would pay for them at negotiated prices. In effect, each DHA would be like a Health Maintenance Organization.

He also stressed that:

> The theory behind such a scheme – which can better be called 'market socialism' than 'privatisation' – is that the managers could then buy services from producers who offered the best value. (Enthoven 1985b)

This concept of the 'internal market' was adopted by most contributors during the debate prior to the publication of *Working for Patients*. For instance, the Kings Fund Institute (1988) described the 'internal market' as having *inter alia* the following features:

> Each district would receive a needs based, per capita allocation. It would be paid for services to outsiders at negotiated prices. It would also control

patient referrals to providers outside the district and would pay for them at negotiated prices.

However, statements from ministers and interpretations in the press, in the months leading up to the publication of *Working for Patients*, appeared to describe a rather different concept of the 'internal market' – a patient-led system. For instance:

the 'internal market', under which GPs could send patients to the health districts with the shortest waiting lists, with the money for their treatment travelling with them. (Brown 1988)

Similar references continued to appear after the publication of *Working for Patients* and this still remains the popular conception of an internal market.

Classification of 'internal markets'

There are then two very different models being described under the heading 'internal market'. Mullen (1989, 1990) characterised them as:

Type I 'Internal Market' Systems
With Type I systems the health authority receives funding for its population; has a specific responsibility for the health/health care of that population; and, in various combinations, provides and/or purchases services from other providers, public or private, to meet the health needs of the population. In the least 'radical' forms, the home authorities remain the main providers of services, but the purchasing of services from other health authorities is increased. In the most 'radical' forms, the home health authority does not provide any services directly, but puts out contracts (with or without competitive tendering) for the entire range of provision. With the Type I 'Internal Market' it is implied, although not always made explicit, that residents of the home health authority may be treated only by 'approved' or 'contracted' providers.

Type II 'Internal Market' Systems
With Type II systems, the health authority receives funding for its population; may be a direct provider of services; but residents can seek treatment anywhere and their home authority is obliged to reimburse the provider. This reimbursement may be either at cost or according to some laid-down scale or negotiated scale or charges. Popularly when this type of 'Internal Market' is mentioned, it is in terms of 'patients being able to shop around to find the shortest waiting list, with their health authority being sent the bill'.

The National Association of Health Authorities described this second model as 'automatic and immediate cross-boundary flow reimbursement', which it stated 'carries the internal market concept to its full fruition, involving transferring the initiative from the planners and treasurers, to the market customers (ie patients) and their advisers (ie GPs) with money following the patient' (NAHA 1988).

Experience from other systems

Some indication of the potential operation of the different types of 'internal market' can be obtained from examining financing and delivery systems elsewhere. The Type II system has many characteristics in common with an insurance-based system, where the insurance company reimburses the provider for care supplied. The Type I system has been likened to a Health Maintenance Organisation (HMO), with the difference that the Health Authority is compulsorily responsible for all residents of a particular location, thus having no choice over membership.

Insurance-based systems

Under most insurance systems, hospitals and health care providers supply services to insured patients and are then reimbursed for the services by the insurer according to either retrospective full-cost reimbursement, or prospective reimbursement.

With retrospective reimbursement schemes, the suppliers of health care receive payment in full from the insurer for all expenditure incurred. Suppliers thus have an incentive to maximise income by encouraging as much activity as possible. They have an incentive to maximise the number of patients treated, maximise the length of stay, maximise the number of surgical procedures performed and the number of diagnostic tests carried out. Such systems are inherently inflationary as they encourage escalation of costs and there is no evidence that they give any encouragement to the cost-effective use of different procedures since the health care suppliers know they will be reimbursed whatever the cost.

In an attempt to control escalating costs, the US Government and insurance companies turned to a prospective payment system – a form of prospective reimbursement. Under this system, health care providers are reimbursed at a predetermined price for each defined unit of workload, regardless of the actual cost involved in providing that unit. The 'unit of workload' can be a day in hospital, a diagnostic test or a particular procedure, but more recently has been in the form of a case. This was associated with the development of Diagnostic Related Groups (DRGs) – a method of 'classifying inpatients into a manageable number of groups, which are both clinically meaningful and homogeneous in resource use' (Culyer and Brazier 1988). Providers are then reimbursed at a set price per case treated, according to the DRG into which the case falls. Prospective payment systems have the advantage that health care suppliers are paid for the amount of work they do and are encouraged to control the cost per case. However, incentives remain for suppliers to treat as many cases as possible; to treat the lowest cost patients within any group; to shift the cost of treatment to other agencies; and to classify patients in the highest cost group possible – known as DRG creep. Thus, with a prospective payment system the funding agency still cannot control total expenditure unless it can control the number of cases. Some insurance companies have attempted to do this by requiring prior approval for treatment.

Health Maintenance Organisations
HMOs were established in the USA in an attempt to control the escalating costs of health care. Instead of health insurance which reimburses the costs of health care on an item-of-service basis, HMOs enrol customers for an annual fee and in return guarantee health care for that year. 'HMOs usually employ their own primary care physicians . . . and either run their own hospital services or buy in from other suppliers' (Culyer and Brazier 1988). Costs are contained and efficiency encouraged since, unlike fee-for-service systems, there is no incentive on the part of the HMO to 'oversupply' services. This is supported by evidence that hospital stays and admission rates are lower in HMOs than under fee-for-service systems (Petchey 1987). However, there have been arguments that the lower costs result from reducing the level of care and jeopardising outcomes, at least to the poorer members (Ware *et al.* 1986). There is an incentive for the HMO to reduce utilisation of services employing, to some extent, general practitioners as gatekeepers. In addition, because HMOs can effectively choose which customers to enrol, there is some suggestion of 'cream skimming', ie HMOs are choosing to enrol lower than average users of services and have an incentive to discriminate against potentially high users of services (Petchey 1987). It must be remembered that the acknowledged success of HMOs in reducing costs should be viewed against the insurance-based systems they replace. The lessons may not have the same applicability in the UK where health care costs are already much lower (Luft 1991).

The White Paper proposals
'Internal markets' and the White Paper

Which model of the 'internal market' was proposed in *Working for Patients* – Type I or Type II? It has been suggested that the rhetoric was Type II, whilst the proposals were Type I, and whilst this may be an oversimplistic observation, it would appear to contain some element of the truth. But what does a more detailed examination of the proposals reveal?

District Health Authorities (DHAs)
The central proposals, ie that DHAs should receive an allocation based on their population and be responsible for providing or acquiring health care services to meet the needs of that population, are fundamentally Type I. However, there are several proposals in *Working for Patients* which introduced elements of a Type II system.

The first is the provision, designed to overcome objections to the loss of GP freedom resultant on the Type I system, that 'DHAs will need to allow for referrals by GPs to hospitals with whom no contracts have been placed, keeping some funds in reserve for this purpose' (DoH 1989a, para. 4.24).

The second Type II provision relates to emergency services. *Working for Patients* gave the assurance that 'the costs of emergency services and those requiring immediate admission to hospital can be met for every patient who needs them, irrespective of whether the patient is resident in a District which has a contract with the hospital (DoH 1989a, para. 4.18). Thus 'if emergency admission as an inpatient is required, the cost should be met by the District of residence. This will require the hospital to levy a charge . . .' (DoH 1989c, para. 2.18).

In respect of both these Type II provisions, 'charges for patients receiving treatment outside their District *and* and outside the scope of its contractual agreements . . . should be recovered direct from the District of residence or from the GP budget holder' (DoH 1989c, para. 2.19).

In addition to such Extra-Contractual Referrals (ECRs), proposals for cost-per-case contracts could also have Type II elements (DoH 1989c). In the absence of controls over referrals by non-fundholding GPs, the provision that under such contracts 'payment would be on a case by case basis, without any prior commitment by either party to the volume of cases which might be so dealt with', would appear very similar to a prospective payment system.

General practitioners as budget holders

General Practitioner Fundholders (GPFHs) with budgets to purchase drugs, outpatient treatment and tests, a limited range of inpatient services and, more recently, community services, are working with an 'internal market' which is mainly Type I. There are some differences from the situation faced by DHAs in that GPFHs are able to choose the population that they serve and are not responsible for the full range of services.

However, GP fundholding does potentially contain some features of a Type II model. In order to control and make best use of their budget, GPFHs must have full knowledge of the cost and scope of the services they are purchasing. However, once the initial referral has been made by the GP the provider, the hospital consultant, makes the diagnosis and determines the treatment (DoH 1989d, para. 3.3). Thus, as the BMA (1989) pointed out, 'these costs would be beyond the control of the general practitioners but could fall on the budget'. Whilst there is no formal provision for GPs to refer their patients for an 'estimate' before deciding whether or not they wish to proceed and pay for treatment, some GPFHs are making referrals 'for opinion only'. However, ethical problems could arise with this and the potential exists for disagreement about the amount and length of treatment, especially for items such as repeat visits to outpatients.

Health care planning and Working for Patients

Against this background, what are the planning roles of the different purchasers and providers?

DHAs

Working for Patients said little about planning but stressed that, having been freed from the obligation actually to provide services:

> ... *DHAs can then concentrate on ensuring that the health needs of the population for which they are responsible are met; that there are effective services for the prevention and control of disease and the promotion of health; that their population has access to a comprehensive range of high quality, value for money services: and on setting targets for and monitoring the performance of those management units for which they continue to have responsibility. (DoH 1989a, para. 2.11)*

The DHA planning role was set out more fully in the guide for Self-Governing Hospitals (NHS Trusts):

> *3.2 Each DHA will have a responsibility to identify the total health care needs of its population and plan how these should be met. It will draw up these plans in the light of national policies and local priorities and resources. It will execute these plans by planning a coordinated series of contracts with selected providers and will then monitor them. The process will necessarily be a dynamic one with DHAs updating their plans annually and modifying their pattern of contracts both to reflect changing needs and to respond to new services becoming available from current or alternative providers. (DoH 1989e)*

The briefing pack accompanying *Working for patients* (DoH 1989h) claimed that at 'Regional and District level planning will be able to respond more effectively to the health needs of the population rather than being tied to details of the operational delivery of services'. However, *Working for Patients* warned that 'Health authority funding will continue to be cash-limited' (DoH 1989a, para. 3.8).

GP fundholders

The planning role of GPFHs is not clear. As noted above, firstly their budgets only cover a limited range of services, and secondly, unlike DHAs, GPFHs can select which patients to take on and thus include in their budget. Therefore, whilst they have a practice planning role, they do not have a population-based planning role. However, the way GPFHs operate could affect planning by their District(s).

Suppliers/providers

The role of providers, ie directly-managed units (DMUs), NHS Trusts and private suppliers, is to deliver 'contracted services within quality and quantity specification to one or a number of clients in return for agreed levels of income' (DoH 1989f). Thus, providers have no formal responsibility to plan to meet the needs of a particular population, but do, of course, need to conduct business planning to secure and fulfil contracts and to attract and treat ECRs.

Health care planning with 'internal markets'

As noted above, elements of both Type I and Type II 'internal markets' appeared in *Working for Patients*. What then are the implications for health care planning of the different types of 'internal market'?

Planning with a Type I 'internal market'

Planning role
Through the placing of contracts, the planning of directly provided services, and control over where its residents may be treated, Type I systems give the home authority the potential to ensure that its priorities are pursued and that the planned balance between health care groups is maintained. Thus with Type I systems, health authorities have considerable potential for health care planning to meet the needs of their populations.

Equality and equity
If health authorities differ in their priorities and make provision for that health care which they consider to be a priority, then Type I systems can mean that residents of different health authorities find access to some forms of health care even more unequal than at present. Other inequalities may result. There is evidence from HMOs that higher income groups gain greater health benefits from the system than do lower income groups (Ware *et al.* 1986). However, another potential source of inequality, 'cream skimming', which arises with HMOs, is removed since, unlike HMOs, DHAs are compulsorily responsible for all residents and thus cannot select only the lower risks. However, DHAs could suffer the secondary effects of such selection if GPFHs select only the lower risks leaving the DHA with the higher-cost patients within any category. DHAs would face the additional challenge of redressing any inequalities resulting from such selection without compensatory funding.

Expenditure control
The very nature of Type I systems means that home authorities have considerable potential for controlling both total expenditure and relative expenditure on different health care groups and types of treatment.

Planning with a Type II 'internal market'

Planning role
With a Type II 'internal market', the home authority would find its health care planning role very restricted with little scope for ensuring

that local needs and priorities are met. This arises because patients are permitted to go anywhere for treatment, leaving the home authority to pay for this treatment, whether or not that authority considers such treatment necessary for that particular patient, whether or not that type of treatment figures in local priorities, and whether or not there are more deserving cases within the authority.

With such a system there seems little to prevent providers behaving in the same way as providers elsewhere where reimbursement systems are in operation. Providers would place no restraint on the services provided or number of cases treated since they would be certain of payment. The home authority, on the other hand, could find its funds being compulsorily diverted to services and cases it considered low priority.

Equality and equity

The Type II model could lead to inequity between health care groups since large amounts of a health authority's budget would be compulsorily diverted to those areas where patients are more mobile and where providers find it most profitable to supply services, ie mainly elective surgery. Other health care groups, especially the so-called priority groups, could lose out. On the other hand, Type II systems could avoid inequalities resulting from differing District priorities, since patients can override local priorities by going elsewhere for treatment. However, new inequalities could arise between patients with the resources and knowledge to seek care outside their district and patients without such resources and/or knowledge.

Overall expenditure control

It is virtually impossible to conceive of a completely Type II system operating successfully with cash-limited health authorities. All experience of retrospective and prospective reimbursement systems points to the difficulties of controlling overall expenditure. Thus, in practice, if a pure Type II system were operating, health authorities would find very large parts of their budgets being compulsorily removed to pay for a much higher consumption of acute (mainly elective surgery) health care, with a consequential diminution of money available for other services.

It can be argued that a fairly radical Type II 'internal market' had already developed in the care of the elderly where much provision is private but much of the funding is public. However, it is debatable how far this model can be extended to the rest of the health service. Firstly, care of the elderly is essentially 'elective'. Secondly, the pre-April 1993 pattern of provision grew up initially on the basis of 'full cost reimbursement' and subsequently on 'prospective payment' – in both cases financed from non-cash-limited public funds. How far would it have developed with cash-limited funds?

Implications in practice

Of course, *Working for Patients* did not advocate a pure Type II model. Indeed, what was advocated was largely Type I. However, the existence of Type II elements, ie both emergency and elective ECRs, gives potential incentives to providers which are very similar to those under insurance-based systems. Unrestricted, the provision for ECRs would mean that providers have every incentive to treat as many patients as possible, in as high a cost category as possible, for 'referrals by GPs to hospitals with whom no contracts have been placed' (DoH 1989a, para. 4.24). Health care providers who do not have a contractual relationship with the home authority would have a financial incentive to over-supply services, in the knowledge that they must be reimbursed. The DHA would find some of its carefully planned resources being diverted to pay for services which may not figure in those plans. Barr *et al.* (1989) went so far as to suggest that 'if the receiving hospital is allowed to "dump" excess capacity by charging no more than short-term marginal cost it will, in effect, be "stealing" part of another District's budget'.

These provisions could clearly lead to the cost-inflationary dangers associated with Type II systems. This point is recognised in an early departure from the principle of GPs' freedom of referral which states that '. . . an open-ended commitment on the part of DHAs to meet all non-contractual referrals would be incompatible with both the disciplines which the new system is intended to inject and with control of budgets (DoH, 1989c, para. 3.3). It is stressed that 'DHAs will need to develop sensitive procedures . . . but will have the right to refuse . . . if there is no satisfactory reason for a distant or expensive referral' (DoH 1989e).

The difficulties in attempting to implement what is basically a Type I system, whilst retaining choice for GPs and patients, were further demonstrated in a more comprehensive description of the proposed provisions for ECRs. Starting from the general principle '. . . that GPs should be free, when necessary, to refer non-emergency cases outside the contract', discussion of the new role of DHAs leads to the conclusion that DHAs cannot 'be put in the position of being a mere cypher and reflecting individual GPs' wishes regardless of their effect on other patient services'. Thus, 'a presumption of the right to make an extra-contractual referral cannot therefore be a guarantee that the DHA would in all cases agree to meet the cost'. Further, a duty is placed on the provider in that 'when a hospital receives an extra-contractual referral, it will need to discuss with the patient's DHA the financial arrangements and other terms . . . (DoH 1989f, paras. 3.14–3.16).

In practice elaborate control mechanisms have been established and

funds for ECRs, both elective and emergency, have been very limited –
an average of only 1.33 per cent of cash limits being allocated initially in
the first year (NAHAT 1991). Most Districts require that each elective
ECR is individually approved, using decision rules for approval of
varying degrees of strictness. For instance, some Districts refuse on
principle to approve elective ECRs where treatment has already started
and some refuse unapproved tertiary referrals (Williamson 1991). Thus,
before any referral is accepted, the hospital must go through a series of
checks to ensure that the patient is covered by a GPFH, by a DHA
contract or by DHA approval for an ECR. This strict control of
ECRs has come under heavy criticism from the Parliamentary Health
Committee (House of Commons 1991) and the DoH has recently
issued new guidance which limits the grounds for refusing ECRs (DoH
1992b).

There are naturally fewer formal controls on emergency ECRs, but
in many cases the dividing line between emergency and non-emergency
is very narrow (Ghodse and Rawaf 1991, Forsythe 1991). There is thus
considerable scope for interpretation over how much treatment can be
considered automatically 'authorised' following emergency admission
and at what point during treatment, if at all, approval must be sought
from the patient's 'home' authority (DoH 1992b).

The effectiveness of health care planning will be strongly influenced
by the strength of the Type II elements in the internal market. Careful
plans could be disrupted if unplanned Type II elements consume a
large part of the DHA's resources. Where the balance will finally lie
is difficult to predict, given the changes in policy emphasis apparent
in only the first two years of operation. However, planning problems
also arise with a Type I system. These concern mainly contracting,
the gatekeeper role, the relationship between DHAs and GPFHs and
rationing.

Contracting
With Type I 'internal markets', some or all the health care services for an
authority's residents are purchased on the basis of contracts. The letting
and operation of such contracts can have a profound effect on health
care planning. Various types of contract can be devised, all of which
contain their own perverse incentives. Two types – block contracts
and cost-and-volume contracts – predominate in the implementation of
Working for Patients. Cost-per-case contracts, as originally proposed,
appear less in evidence possibly because of their Type II nature described
above. With population-based block contracts, ie contracts to provide
a defined population with its full requirements for a specified range
of services, providers have an incentive to treat as few patients as
possible, to undersupply and to reduce the level of service to the
minimum specified in the contract. With cost-and-volume contracts,
which specify the number of cases to be treated, the provider has an
incentive to select the cheaper cases within the categories specified and
to minimise the level of service per patient. In all contracts there is an

incentive to shift the costs on to other services outside that contract, for instance, from hospital care to community care.

Further problems arise from the creation of 'packages' of services or care, a corollary of contracting and tendering for services. Much of the debate on the 'internal market' appeared to relate to elective surgery, which lends itself to 'packages' of care. It is easy to grasp the concept of tendering for the oft-quoted '200 hip replacements' and, apart from dangers such as 'cream skimming', this appears relatively non-problematic. However, *Working for Patients* proposed putting the entire health service out to tender – in discrete parcels. How a contract could be agreed for, say, general medicine, other than on a population basis is difficult to envisage. If the contract is made for, say, 100 pneumonia cases, or for 100 fractures (or 100 births!), what happens to the 101st case that comes along? Basically, the choice of contract raises the fundamental question of 'which party carries the risk?' With block contracts providers carry the risk of catering for unplanned increases in demand and in effect accept open-ended contracts at fixed prices. With cost-and-volume contracts, the risk is carried by purchasers who have to provide additional funds if demand exceeds planned levels. Thus, a Type I 'internal market' needs a mixture of types of contracts, including population-based block contracts. However, the latter are unattractive to providers.

Other problems could arise as a result of contracting. Firstly, what is the position of a health authority which, having identified a need for a particular service, cannot find a provider? This could prove to be a particular problem for DHAs left without any relevant DMUs. Secondly, individual providers enter the 'internal market' with different historical endowments of facilities and are unlikely to be able to compete equally for contracts. Thirdly, problems might arise from the interdependence of services. Is it really possible to 'contract-out' some specialties and still retain a comprehensive service? Fourthly, annual contracting poses planning problems for providers. They will need far longer commitment to feel confident in developing new services.

The gatekeeper role
Whilst the home authority can plan and contract for the services it identifies as being required to meet the needs of its population, it is not clear who decides which individuals will receive those services. In other words, which party, the purchaser or the provider, determines which patients shall be treated on the contract? If it is left to the provider there are strong incentives to select the lower cost, least complicated cases, within the contracted category.

The Department of Health (1989f) proposed that 'as a minimum, the contracting parties should consider specifying: . . . the criteria for admission and discharge of inpatients and for day/outpatient referrals'. However, it is difficult to see how such criteria can be formulated to ensure that treatment is received by those individuals that the home authority would have chosen.

Lilford (1989) saw the ability of the home authority to choose who receives treatment as a major benefit of the new system, stating that 'some patients will still go without treatment, but commissioning agents will help patients with the greatest need or best prognosis. Therefore, instead of the budget running out, say, after nine months of the year, the commissioner will preselect for the greatest perceived need'. However, Lilford gave no indication as to how this preselection might work.

Some HMOs 'employ' GPs to act as gatekeepers, and currently in the NHS GPs act as the initial gatekeeper to secondary care, with consultants and other hospital doctors acting as the final gatekeeper. It is not clear, with funding split from the provision of services, whether this system will continue to work in compliance with the plans of the home authority. GPs are neither employees nor agents of the home authority and have no contractual, and little moral, duty to act as the authority's gatekeepers. Indeed, since GPs will feel that their primary duty is to their own patients, there is no incentive to attempt to limit their patients' share of the contracts. Hospital doctors are the agents of the provider, not the purchasing authority, and again cannot be expected automatically to take on the gatekeeper role. Some DHAs via their Directors of Public Health are addressing this problem by agreeing admission and treatment protocols with consultants working for their contracted providers.

GP fundholding overcomes the gatekeeper problem since the GPs act as gatekeepers to their own budgets. However, if GPs were given budgets for the whole range of patient care, as in one of the alternatives suggested by Maynard (1986), various problems could arise including incentives to undersupply, especially if GPs were permitted to retain budgetary savings. Bevan (1984, 1989) avoids this particular problem in proposing a simulated HMO based on GPs' choices. Under this 'simulated market', districts would receive a population-based allocation and would pass this allocation 'down to GPs in the form of notional budgets for hospital and community health services; GPs would exercise choice, as in the model of Maynard *et al;* but that choice would be made against the notional budget, where GPs stand neither to lose nor to gain financially from how their actual use of services compared with their budget' (Bevan 1989).

Coexistence of DHAs and GPFHs
Although DHAs and GPFHs both face a largely Type I internal market, their coexistence raises some planning issues. As noted above, whereas DHAs are explicitly responsible for meeting the needs of defined geographical populations, GPFHs are concerned only with the needs of their registered patients. The ability of DHAs to plan for their populations can be constrained if substantial proportions of their population-based allocations are diverted to GPFHs, who may not share the planning priorities of the DHA. To help overcome this problem, some DHAs are attempting to involve GPFHs in the

planning process. Even with such collaboration, DHAs have faced problems resulting from the different budget levels set for GPFHs. In the first year of operation these budgets were established largely on the basis of the imputed expenditure of the practice in the previous year, resulting in very great differences in funding per registered patient (Day and Klein 1991). However, even when the question of budget setting has been resolved, the incentive for GPFHs to select lower risk patients (Scheffler 1989) could leave DHAs responsible for the higher risk patients, without commensurate funding. Indeed, there may prove to be some 'natural' GPFH selection against higher risk patients, since such practices are less likely to be found in inner cities (Drummond *et al.* 1990, Dyson 1992).

Rationing

An advantage of the Type I model is that it enables the DHA to determine its priorities and plan to ensure that the needs of its population are met. However, the more explicit regime brought about by the purchaser–provider split has led to increased interest in explicit rationing, where DHAs identify treatments they will not fund. Such explicit rationing, which must be compared with the alternative of rationing by clinical judgement and waiting lists, can appear very attractive. However, proposals which explicitly exclude whole categories of treatments and conditions appear to make no allowance for variation in severity within any condition group. Thus, whilst on average one treatment may have a lower cost-benefit ratio than another, this may not be true of cases at the margin. Further, if waiting is used as part of the rationing system, patients at least have a choice between waiting, with zero direct money price, and not waiting, by paying for private treatment. If some classes of treatment are completely excluded, those unable to opt for private treatment also lose the option of waiting. Finally, can a national health system coexist with the freedom for individual local health authorities to exclude treatments which other authorities include?

Some DHAs are setting priorities by limiting the number of certain types of treatment they will purchase – using protocols to attempt to ensure those treatments are received by the highest priority patients. However, there are some indications that such 'soft' rationing is considered insufficiently rigorous for the new NHS, and that DHAs must face up to the necessity of rationing by excluding whole classes of treatment (Klein and Redmayne 1992, Millar 1992).

Markets and planning

The 'market' proposals in *Working for Patients* can have other implications for health care planning, irrespective of the relative strengths of the Type I and Type II models. Many of these relate to the characteristics of the health care services that can be obtained to

meet the needs of the population identified by the planning authority
– the DHA.

Volume of services

Many of the benefits intended to flow from *Working for Patients*
appeared to be predicated on the assumption of an increase in the total
volume of services provided. This was made explicit in an executive
letter which stated that the 'objective of increasing the efficiency of the
NHS will only be realised if competition delivers more in the value of
savings and/or quality improvements than it adds to transaction costs'
(DoH 1989g).

Thus, it was hoped that greater efficiency would achieve a higher
volume of services. There is evidence from the US that 'substantial
savings are achievable through the transfer of services from low volume,
high cost, low efficiency centres'. On the strength of this Petchey (1989)
concludes that 'there is the potential for some cost saving even if we are
unable to begin to quantify it'. However, there are countervailing forces
which might result in a lower volume of services.

Firstly, there are increased transaction costs and more staff are
required just to work the new system. The commentary to the Bill
to effect the proposals estimated a permanent increase of about 3500
staff, in addition to short-term increases in staff (HMSO 1989).

Secondly, there is a risk that higher prices charged by monopoly
suppliers will result in DHAs being able to purchase a lower volume of
services than provided at present. As Barr *et al.* (1989) put it, 'We must
expect the new independent hospitals to act like any profit-maximizing
firm. They will attempt to differentiate their products. Having many
expensive specialist facilities this will not be difficult. We would expect
them to corner discrete specialist areas of care and charge monopoly
rent for the cases they treat. There will be no effective competition'.
To counter this danger one of the Working Papers stated that '. . . the
Secretary of State will need reserve powers to prevent a self-governing
hospital with anything near to a monopoly of service provision from
exploiting its position, for example by charging unreasonably high
prices for its services' (DoH 1989b, para. 2.15). However, NHS Trusts
have power to fix pay levels and few have suggested that this will result
in a general fall in pay – indeed a general increase in pay levels has
been anticipated in an attempt to attract scarce staff (Maynard 1989).
Much of the scope for pay reduction within the NHS has already
been exploited in the competitive tendering for support services. Unless
entirely compensated by increased efficiency increased costs will result
in increased prices and thus lower volumes.

Thirdly, a possible source of reduced volumes lies in the dividing up
of services for the purpose of contracting. Many services offered by
health providers can be considered as joint products. Thus it is possible
that, as a result of letting out contracts for individual services possibly to
different suppliers, the aggregate cost of the individual contracts (each

of which would have to be independently viable) would exceed the combined cost of the original integrated services. Alternatively a lower volume of services would be secured for the same cost.

Fourthly, drawing on US experience, Light (1991a & b) suggests that competition itself may lead to lower efficiency and increased costs.

Waiting for services

One of the stated aims of *Working for Patients* was the reduction in waiting time for treatment. Indeed, one criterion for placing contracts and monitoring providers is the length of waiting lists and the delay in treatment. However, it is possible that the rationing function of waiting lists will simply be moved to an earlier stage in the treatment cycle. A provider, being judged on the length of waiting lists, will simply accept for treatment the number of cases provided for in the contract, quite properly refusing further cases unless reimbursed on a cost-per-case basis. Indeed, there is anecdotal evidence of this happening already (Mullen 1992). Refused cases will not appear on the waiting list. Further, by controlling the rate of acceptances for treatment, it will be possible for providers to guarantee immediate treatment for those accepted.

Balance of services

Differential increases in prices might cause problems for planning by causing imbalances. Indeed for some treatments there may be no service available since the providers consider it unprofitable. Markets imply a willing seller and a willing buyer.

Location of services

The proposals, both Type I and Type II, involve 'purchasing' services, possibly at a considerable distance. This could lead to problems for a DHA in planning equitable, integrated and accessible services for its resident population. Studies have shown that a proportion of patients are willing to travel to receive elective surgery more speedily, but there is little evidence on this question in relation to other services. For instance Lister (1988) asked: 'what comfort would it be for elderly and severely ill patients to hear of "competitive" NHS hospitals with vacant beds in Liverpool or Devon?' Culyer *et al.* (1988) stressed that 'care will have to be exercised to ensure that very sick and elderly patients are not treated or cared for long distances away from their homes and families'. Brotherton and Harris (1988) point to increased difficulties in arranging back-up services and in discharging patients into community health services, if hospital services have been provided far from their home locations.

Type of services provided

It is noted above that the main planning focus for providers is business planning to enable them to secure and fulfil contracts. Except in those cases where contracts are population-based, which exist although not officially envisaged in the post-review NHS, providers have responsibility only for those patients they treat and have no responsibility for a particular population. As Troop and Zimmern (1989) express it, 'at the hospital or service end the objective is entirely different. Its aim is efficient and effective service provision. It is the "provider" of services. Its unit of concern is not the population but the patient episode and a well run hospital will know exactly, for each category of patient, the cost of care and its outcome'.

In the past some clinicians have been criticised for being concerned only with the patients they actually see and not with the wider population. As a result, considerable effort has gone into attempting to relate individual clinical decisions and actions to wider health and resource issues. However, the introduction of proposals which structurally divorce the providers of services from wider population considerations, may be considered by some to be a retrograde step and, in practice, may affect the type of care delivered.

Locality planning

Over recent years there have been various developments in health care planning with the aim of better meeting the needs of particular populations. One such development is Locality Planning, which aims to plan integrated services for a community at a more local level than the District. How such planning is faring within the post-review NHS is not fully clear. There is some interest in locality purchasing, with schemes ranging from local input into DHA purchasing decisions, to total devolution of resources to locality teams for them to secure the services required. However, such schemes raise questions not only of the availability of the necessary expertise for contracting at a local level, but the more problematic question of how large a population is required to act as a 'risk-pool' for different services.

Philosophy of health and health care

The underlying philosophy of health and health care provision has a profound influence on the nature and achievements of health care planning. This is a major area which can only be touched on here.

The emphasis on *Working for Patients* on services to individual patients, provisions such as 'Life-Style Consultations' in connection with the 1990 Contract for GPs, and the introduction of the Patient's

Charter (DoH 1991), can be viewed as a reinforcement of the individual-istic view of health. This view has come under criticism from some commentators (Navarro 1976, Doyal 1979) since, they claim, it leads to treating the causes of ill-health as being individual, requiring individually orientated therapeutic responses or prevention through individuals changing their own way of life. Thus, it is claimed, the economic and political environment is absolved from responsibility for disease and collective responses are rendered unnecessary. Whether *The Health of the Nation* will counteract this individualist bias will depend on the manner of its implementation (DoH 1992a).

Another related factor is the move towards treating health care provision as a tradeable commodity. Navarro (1986) claims that 'capitalism attempts to replace services pure and simple with com-modities that can be bought and sold on the private market' and rather more strongly, Waitzkin (1983) suggests that 'from the standpoint of potential profit, there is no reason that corporations should view medical products differently from other products. The commodification of health care and its associated technology is a necessary feature of the capitalist political–economic system.'

Conclusions

With the implementation of the *Working for Patients* proposals, the planning roles of the various parts of the NHS have changed considerably and have become more differentiated. The planning role of providers, whether DMUs, NHS Trusts or the private sector, largely revolves around business planning to secure and fulfil contracts. Population-based planning relating to identifying the needs of a population and ensuring these needs are met – generally to promote the health of a defined population – is the province of Health Authorities.

The resource allocation proposals in *Working for Patients*, ie weighted population funding for Regions and Districts, without compensation for cross-boundary flows should, despite considerable misgivings about the methodology employed, assist Districts in their planning role. However, the separation of funding from the provision of services – the 'internal market' – could prove more problematic for planning. Two distinct types of 'internal market' have been identified, both of which have considerable implications for population-based planning, for the pursuit of priorities, and for equity and equality whether between geographical areas, social groups or health care groups. Both types of 'internal market' were present in *Working for Patients* and there is evidence of tension between the two types of provision. The eventual outcome for planning to meet needs, to secure equity and to maximise health, will depend very much on the relative strengths, in practice, of the two types of 'internal market'.

References

Barr, N, Glennerster, H and le Grand, J (1989) 'Working for patients? The right approach?' *Social Policy and Administration* 23 2, 117–127

Bevan, G (1984), 'Organising the finance of hospitals by simulated markets' *Fiscal Studies* 5, 44–62

Bevan, G (1989), 'Reforming UK health care: internal markets of emergent planning?' *Fiscal Studies* 10 1 53–71

Bevan, G and Brazier, J (1987) 'Financial incentives of subregional RAWP', *British Medical Journal* 295, 3 October 1987, 836–838

BMA (1989) *Special Report of the Council of the British Medical Association on the Government's White Paper "Working for Patients"'* SRM2, British Medical Association

Brazier, J (1986) 'Is cross-charging the solution to the problem of cross boundary flows?', 26–42 in *Reviewing RAWP*, Social Medicine and Health Services Research Unit, Guy's and St Thomas's Hospitals, London

Brazier, J (1987) 'Accounting for cross boundary flows' *British Medical Journal* 295, 10 October 1987, 898–900

Brotherton, P and Harris, R (1988) *Their Hands in Our Safe* Socialist Health Association, p. 7

Brown, C (1988) 'Internal market could lead to hospital closures' *Independent* 9 July 1988

Cooper, MH and Culyer, AJ (1970) 'An economic assessment of some aspects of the operation of the National Health Service', Appendix A, 187–250 in *Health Services Financing* British Medical Association

Culyer, AJ and Brazier, JE (1988) *'Alternatives for organising the provision of health services in the UK*, IHSM Working Paper No. 4 on Alternative Delivery and Funding for Health Care

Culyer, AJ, Brazier, JE and O'Donnell, OO (1988) *'Organising health service provision: drawing on experience'*, IHSM Working Paper No. 5 on Alternative Delivery and Funding for Health Care

Day, P and Klein, R (1991) 'Variations in budgets of fundholding practices' *British Medical Journal* 303, 6775, 168–170

DoH (1989a) *Working for Patients* White Paper on the NHS, Cmd 555, HMSO, London

DoH (1989b) *Self-Governing Hospitals* NHS Review Working Paper 1, HMSO, London

DoH (1989c) *Funding and Contracts for Hospital Services* NHS Review Working Paper 2, HMSO, London

DoH (1989d) *Practice Budgets for General Medical Practitioners* NHS Review Working Paper 3, HMSO, London

DoH (1989e) *Self-governing Hospitals: An initial guide* HMSO, London

DoH (1989f) *Contracts for Health Services: Operational Principles* HMSO, London

DoH (1989g) *Implementing the White Paper: Discussion Document on Pricing and Openness in Contracts for Health Services* EL(89)MB/171

DoH (1989h) *NHS Review: Briefing Pack for NHS Managers* DoH, London

DoH (1991) *The Patients Charter* Department of Health, London

DoH (1992a) *The Health of the Nation* Cmd 1896, HMSO, London

DoH (1992b) *Guidance on Extra Contractual Referrals* issued under EL(92)60, Department of Health, London

DHSS (1970) Circular 3/70 to Regional Hospital Board Chairmen, London

DHSS (1972) *Management Arrangements for the Reorganised National Health Service* HMSO, London

DHSS (1976) *Sharing Resources for Health in England: Report of the Resource Allocation Working Party* HMSO, London

Doyal, L (1979) *The Political Economy of Health* Pluto Press

Drummond, MF, Crump, B, Hawkes, R and Marchment, M (1990) 'General practice fundholding' *British Medical Journal* **301**, 5764, 1288–1289

Dyson, R (1992) quoted by MacLachlan, R in 'report of the First Annual Conference of the National Association of Fundholding Practices' *The Health Service Journal* **102**, 5333, 15

Enthoven, AC (1985a) *Reflections on the Management of the National Health Service* NPHT

Enthoven, AC (1985b) 'National Health Service: Some reforms that might be politically feasible' *The Economist* **295**, 7399, 19–22

Forsythe, M (1991) 'Extracontractual referrals: the story so far' *British Medical Journal* **303**, 6801, 470–480

Ghodse, B and Rawaf, S (1991) 'Extracontractual referrals in the first three months of NHS reforms' *British Medical Journal* **303**, 6801, 497–499

HMSO (1989) *National Health Service and Community Care Bill* 50/3, HMSO, London

House of Commons (1991) *Public Expenditure on Health Services and Personal Social Services* Parliament, House of Commons Health Committee, 3rd Report, Vol. 1, Report 614–1, 17 July 1991

Kings Fund Institute (1988) *Health Finance: Assessing the Options* Briefing Paper No. 4, London

Klein, R and Redmayne, S (1992) *Patterns of Priorities: a study of the purchasing and rationing policies of the health authorities* NAHAT Research Paper No. 7, National Association of Health Authorities, Birmingham

Light, DW (1991a) 'Perestroika for Britain's NHS' *The Lancet* **337**, 778–779

Light, DW (1991b) 'Observations on the NHS reforms: an American perspective' *British Medical Journal* **303**, 6802, 568–570

Lilford, R (1989) 'Looking to a better future' *The Health Service Journal* **28**, September 1989, 1190–1191

Lister, J (ed.) (1988) *Cutting the Lifeline: The Fight for the NHS* Journeyman

Luft, HS (1991) 'Translating the US HMO experience to other health systems' *Health Affairs* **10**, 3, 172–186

Maynard, A (1986) 'Performance incentives in general practice' in Teeling Smith, G (ed.) *Health, Education and General Practice* OHE, London, 44–46

Maynard, A (1989) *Whither the National Health Service* NHS White Paper Occasional paper 1, Centre for Health Economics, University of York

Mays, N (1989) 'NHS resource allocation after the 1989 White Paper: a critique of the research for the RAWP Review' *Community Medicine* **11**, 3, 173–186

Mays, N and Bevan, G (1987) *Resource Allocation in the Health Service* Occasional Papers on Social Administration No. 81, Bedford Square Press

Millar B (1992) 'Irrational behaviour' *The Health Service Journal* **102**, 5329, 14–15

MoH (1962) *A Hospital Plan for England and Wales* Cmd 1604, HMSO, London

Mullen, PM (1978) *RAWP and Resource Allocation in the NHS* HSMC Discussion Paper Series No. 13, University of Birmingham

Mullen, PM (1986) 'Funding of supra-authority services' *Public Money* **6**, 2, 55–58

Mullen, PM (1989) *Health and the Internal Market: Implications of the White Paper* Discussion paper No. 25, Health Services Management Centre, University of Birmingham

Mullen, PM (1990) 'Which internal market? The NHS White Paper and internal markets' *Financial Accountability and Management* **6**, 1, 33–50

Mullen, PM (1992) *Waiting Lists and the NHS Review: Reality and Myths* Research Report 29, Health Services Management Centre, University of Birmingham

NAHA (1988) *Funding the NHS: Which Way forward?* A NAHA Consultation Document, National Association of Health Authorities

NAHAT (1991) *Spring Financial Survey 1991* National Association of Health Authorities and Trusts, Birmingham

Navarro, V (1976) *Medicine Under Capitalism* Croom Helm

Navarro, V (1986) *Crisis, Health, and Medicine* Tavistock Publications

Petchey, R (1987) 'Health maintenance organisations: Just what the doctor ordered?' *Journal of Social Policy* **16**, 4, 489–507

Petchey, R (1989) 'The politics of destabilisation' *Critical Social Policy* **9**, 1, 82–97

Scheffler, R (1989) 'Adverse selection: the Achilles heel of the NHS reforms' *The Lancet* **I**, 8644, 950–952

Troop, P and Zimmern, R (1989) 'A model for the post-White Paper NHS' *NHS Management Bulletin* July 1989, 23, 4–5

Waitzkin, H (1983) 'A Marxist view of health and health care' in Mechanic, D (ed.) *Handbook of Health, Health Care and the Health Professions* The Free Press, 657–682

Ware, JE *et al.* (1986) 'Comparison of health outcomes at a health maintenance organisation with those of fee-for-service care' *The Lancet* i, No. 8488, 1017–1022

Williamson, JD (1991) 'Dealing with extracontractual referrals' *British Medical Journal* 303, 6801, 499–504

3 The NHS reforms and the finance function

Tony Cook

Introduction

Like many other aspects of the National Health Service, the finance function has changed and is continuing to change over time. In recent years that pace of change has been particularly rapid. The chapter aims to assess the NHS reforms in the light of the changing nature of the finance function.

It will consider first of all the state of the finance function as it stood at the end of 1988, and assess what changes had recently taken place, what were in progress and what further developments could logically have been anticipated.

In that context we will then turn to the reforms and consider how they affect, specifically, accounting and finance. We will examine the financial aims and objectives, how they impact on the finance function, some of the problems of implementation and whether they are consistent with the changes already in hand. Finally some conclusions are drawn as to the desirability of the changes initiated in the legislation.

It is also important to note, at the outset, the distinction between *financial* accounting and *management* accounting. Financial accounting concerns the need to have systems in place which ensure that financial transactions (such as the payment of wages) are properly conducted and that appropriate records are maintained. Management accounting is concerned with ensuring that appropriate financial information is provided to the management of the organisation to ensure that they can manage it as well as possible and (in the public sector) deliver the greatest value for money.

The developing finance function before *Working for Patients*

Figure 3.1 is a familiar, and a very useful one for explaining the financial structure of the NHS *in England*. It was first published by

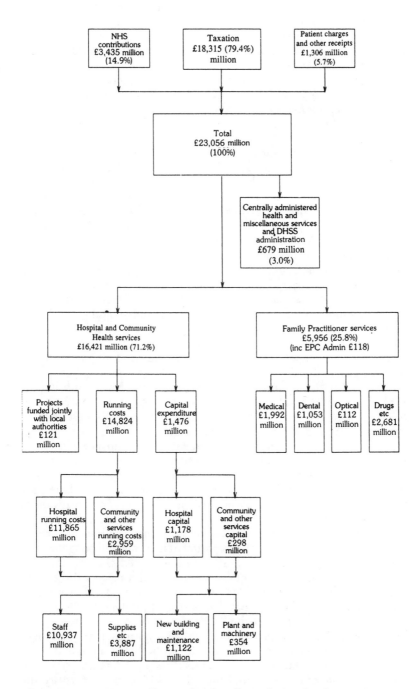

Figure 3.1 NHS Funding and expenditure in England, 1990/91

the Department of Health in 1983, and was then updated in successive Annual Reports of the NHS in England (DHSS 1986). However it has not officially been published for the last few years and the figures shown for 1990/91 are unofficial ones culled from the published NHS Annual Accounts (DHSS 1992).

The figure shows the nature of expenditure (hospital running costs, capital expenditure, general practice expenditure) and shows clearly the split which existed between the Hospital and Community Health Services (on the left of the figure) and the Family Practitioner Services (on the right).

Figure 3.1a is a variant of Figure 3.1 in which the *organisations* responsible for committing expenditure are shown. Thus on the right-hand side there is a box for the Family Practitioner Committees (FPCs) which were responsible for making payments to the practitioners. On the left there are boxes under both 'running costs' and 'capital expenditure' for Regional Health Authorities (RHAs), District Health Authorities (DHAs) and Units. Note the relative sizes of the boxes. Under 'running costs' there is a small box for RHAs and a large box for DHAs indicating that the bulk of expenditure is actually incurred by the District Health Authorities. Under 'capital expenditure' the situation is reversed as it is the Regional Health Authorities who are responsible for planning, designing and building the major capital schemes. In both cases Units are shown as 'dotted line' boxes indicating that very little expenditure is actually paid for by the Units even though, of course, they are where the bulk of resources are deployed.

Figure 3.2 is also familiar. It originates from the Korner 6th Report (NHS/DHSS 1984) and shows how money is spent in a hospital day by day. Note the three levels of expenditure analysis described as 'subjective', 'departmental' and 'patient care'.

Let us consider the ongoing development of NHS finance within this framework. Prior to 1974, hospital accounts were generally maintained only on the traditional income and expenditure account basis which showed only a 'subjective' analysis of expenditure (ie salaries for doctors, salaries for nurses, expenditure on drugs etc). This corresponds to level 1 in Figure 3.2.

Following the 1974 NHS reorganisation we had the introduction of what is now referred to as the departmental system of budgeting (as in level 2 in Figure 3.2). While it has been refined and improved in several respects this departmental system of budgeting is still the main tool of financial management on the vast majority of NHS hospital sites. Moreover, as Maynard has demonstrated (Maynard 1984), it has proved to be effective in enabling Health Authorities to live within their means. Recent cases where Health Authorities have overspent have usually stemmed from a failure to properly install and operate such a system. In value for money terms if the only financial objective is the achievement of 'economy' then the NHS is well served by the basic departmental system of budgeting.

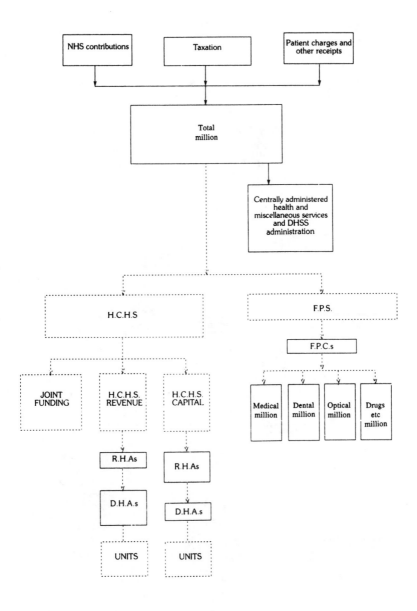

Figure 3.1a   NHS funding and expenditure in England

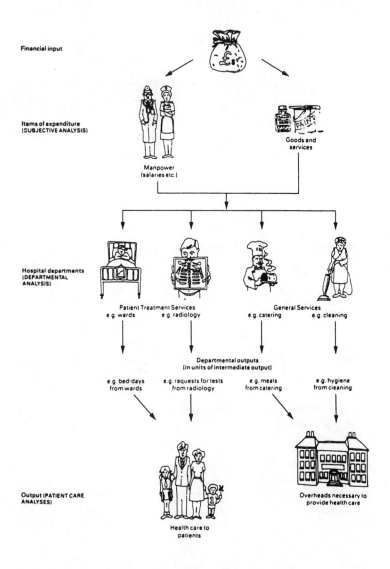

Figure 3.2   How money is used in a hospital day by day

However we need to address the wider issues of VFM. If we accept the 'three Es' definition of VFM – economy, efficiency and effectiveness – then financial information systems need to be developed which will promote 'efficiency' and 'effectiveness' in addition to economy. It is in this wider context that the departmental system of budgeting becomes inadequate. In particular it is subject to three well documented limitations. They are:

1 It provides no analysis of expenditure by health care category – however defined. Thus, for example, if we wished to know how much we are spending on orthopaedic surgery the departmental analysis of expenditure will not tell us. This is because part of that expenditure is incurred in the operating theatres, part in the wards, part in the X-ray department etc. However, the departmental system of budgeting contains no mechanism to identify those individual parts, nor any mechanism to bring them together to give a total for orthopaedic surgery. This limitation is crucial, of course, to our ability to plan expenditure in health care terms.

2 Doctors – in discharging their clinical duties – make decisions which commit resources for which they are not the budget holders. Thus when a doctor asks for an X-ray or path lab test, or prescribes drugs, or decides that a patient should remain in hospital for a further two days, he is making a financial as well as a clinical decision. However he is not presumed to be financially accountable for such decisions.

3 The corollary to point 2 is that it is budget holders – such as the chief pharmacist or chief pathologist – who are expected to manage their departments within a predetermined budget, although the level of activity in their departments is outside their control. The chief pharmacist, for example, has no control over the number of prescriptions that come into his department. However, he cannot refuse to dispense a prescription on the grounds that to do so would make him overspend against his budget.

Knowledge of these limitations is not new. The Royal Commission Report of 1978 (Royal Commission on the NHS 1978) identified them, and the last decade has seen several initiatives to develop improved financial information and to overcome them.

All of these initiatives share the common approach of adding an additional – clinical – analysis of hospital expenditure. We can, therefore, conceive of a simple three dimensional model (Figure 3.3).

Clearly as with the existing 'subjective' and 'departmental' analyses so the clinical analysis of expenditure may be provided in greater or lesser degrees of detail. Conventional wisdom – as illustrated for example in the Korner 6th Report – has come to identify five possible levels of analysis for the clinical axis:

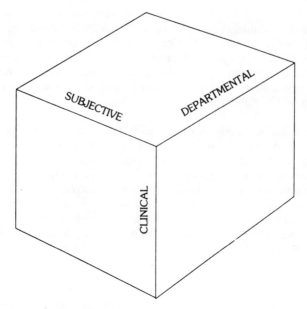

Figure 3.3 Three dimensional model

1 *to client group* (mental handicap, maternity, the elderly etc);

2 *to clinical specialty* (orthopaedics, paediatrics, obstetrics etc);

3 *to consultant* (and his clinical team);

4 *by disease category* (hip replacements, appendicectomies, strokes etc);

5 *to the individual patient.*

In fact attention has been paid at different times and in different initiatives to developing financial information appropriate to each of the above levels of analysis.

For example, analyses of expenditure to *client group* have been available at the national level since the mid-1970s. These have been calculated by a technique misleadingly known as '*programme budgeting*'. This involves making very broad brush assumptions about how costs can be allocated to broadly defined client groups. Such figures are of limited value in that they contain no guide as to whether the resources have been spent efficiently or effectively. Likewise the title is misleading in that it is not a true budgeting system. Nevertheless, limited though their value may be, the NHS in England has not made consistent use of programme budget figures (unlike in Scotland where the Health Boards have produced historical and projected figures to assist health care planning).

From the 1987/88 financial year, Health Authorities have been required to produce '*specialty costs*'. These are, by definition, calculations of average costs per case at *specialty* level, prepared at the end of each financial year on historical bases. The technique has been existing for some years, and should provide information which may be of use in identifying high levels of expenditure within a particular specialty within a District, and should be of value in assisting local planning.

If we can now move down the clinical axis to level 5 – that of the *individual patient* – there have been various trials in techniques of *patient costing*; designed by definition, to calculate the cost of treating each patient. Of particular interest here is the work of the Financial Information Project which has been in existence since 1979. There are arguments in favour of analysing costs down to the individual patient. However it should be recognised that while it is possible to analyse costs retrospectively to the individual patient, it is not possible to plan prospectively to the individual patient. It is not possible for example to predict that Mr Smith will have a heart attack or that Mrs Williams will fall over in the snow and break her leg. We cannot budget down to the level of the individual patient.

Thus all three of these techniques, programme budgeting, specialty costing and patient costing, are of some value but do not overcome all the limitations of departmental budgets.

Consequently recent developments have concentrated upon what may be described as systems of 'clinical budgeting'. In the UK there have been three initiatives of note, and variants have concentrated on three levels – specialty, consultant and disease category – in our clinical analysis. These three initiatives are CASPE, 'management budgeting' and 'resource management'.

CASPE – an acronym for clinical and service planning evaluation – is a small research group based at the King's Fund College. It was also established in 1979 and has developed systems of clinical budgeting – perhaps with varying degrees of success – at a small number of NHS hospitals. A key feature of the CASPE approach has been the emphasis on the *planning* rather than the *control* aspect of budgeting through PACTs (planning agreements with clinical teams). Discussions were held with consultants and agreements drawn up as to what would be the expected workload for the clinical team and what resources they may require to process that workload. The early CASPE trials were actually discrete information systems developed with little finance department involvement. In such cases the District Treasurer would have argued that financial control over the hospital remained with the traditional departmental budgets.

The development of 'management budgeting' was one of the recommendations of the Griffiths Report of 1983. In a supporting paper Blyth (1983) argued that the objective was 'to develop management budgets involving clinicians at unit level with the emphasis on management rather than accountancy. The aim is to produce an unsophisticated system in which workload related budgets covering financial and manpower allocations and full overhead costs are closely related to workable service objectives, against which performance and progress can be compared'.

That is the key paragraph in a paper which logically argued the case for a better budgeting system and set out a number of principles on which it should be based. By and large those principles were soundly based although one could take issue with the question of 'full overhead costs'. This does not follow what is generally accepted as good industrial/commercial practice. The paragraph also contains a clue as to why management budgeting has been perceived, by some, to be a failure in that it talks of an 'unsophisticated system'. It *is* possible to have a system which includes 'workload related budgets concerning financial and manpower allocations etc' but it is not going to be 'unsophisticated'. In that respect Blyth was unrealistically optimistic. Nevertheless the overall principle is important. There *is* a need for workload related budgets covering financial and manpower allocations, related to workable service objectives, against which performance and progress can be compared.

In the light of Griffiths the DoH funded four 'demonstration districts'. These too have had their successes and failures. They have demonstrated that it *is* possible to construct systems of clinical budgeting in acute hospitals. However, they have also thrown up a number of problems. The need to have adequate supporting information systems in such key areas as patient administration, radiography, pharmacy and pathology is one of the technical problems. Even more important however are the organisational and behavioural issues: what are the correct managerial relationships between the medical, nursing and paramedical professions? Above all to what extent can clinicians be persuaded to accept that they are financially and managerially accountable for their decisions? And if they do, how should their organisational structure be incorporated into the managerial hierarchy of the hospital? Insofar as management budgeting was seen to be a failure it was because it was perceived to be too much of a finance-led exercise which did not adequately tackle the organisational and behavioural issues.

Hence we had the move, in 1986, to 'resource management'. HN (86)34 (DHSS 1986) initiated the change of title and the very real change of emphasis. It identified four lessons which had been learned from the management budgeting experience:

1 Doctors and nurses need to be centrally involved in management arrangements.

2 Doctors and nurses need to be centrally involved in specifying the information requirements of the new systems.

3 Effective financial management support is vital.

4 The pace at which management budgets are introduced will need to be carefully judged.

Six acute hospitals were identified to be pilot sites for the RMI. From a narrow accounting point of view the significant change was that they were to be geared to the introduction of patient 'case-mix planning and costing'. Such a system requires that patients suffering from similar diseases and requiring similar treatment regimes should be grouped together. The budgeting system then becomes capable of reflecting the complexity of cases handled, rather than the simple numbers of patients treated. In terms of our levels of analysis on the clinical axis we are now moving from level 3, consultant, to level 4, disease category. Although still in its infancy, there have already been several approaches to case mix accounting.

For example at Southmead – one of the original management budgeting demonstration districts – the approach was to ask each of the participating consultants to define the 10 or 12 case types which probably made up 80 to 90 per cent of their regular workload. For each of those case types a treatment pattern was identified and costs applied in order to build up a treatment cost for the typical patient. Such an approach is perfectly logical from a local management accounting point of view. However, it suffers from the drawback that each consultant is defining his own case type and will do it differently from another consultant in another hospital. It therefore makes comparisons difficult.

Internationally the most widely used approach is based on the international disease classification developed at Yale University. Under this approach all acute patients can be allocated to one of 475 Diagnosis Related Groups (DRGs). Already this system has been extensively used in the USA where increasingly the Medicare system is reimbursing hospitals on the basis of a price per DRG. In the UK all of the new resource management sites initially based their development of case-mix accounting on DRGs, although more recently they have been developing an improved British classification known as HRGs (Healthcare Resource Groups).

Yet another American approach is being developed at John Hopkins University. This recognises that even within the same disease category some patients are more severely ill than others and require correspondingly more extensive – and more expensive – treatments. This approach therefore introduces severity ratings whereby patients' illnesss are then classified into one of four categories of severity, within the same disease category.

It should be recognised that we are still in the early days of case mix accounting. Moreover difficulties arise, simply, because we are dealing with patients in a hospital rather than products in a factory. Inevitably therefore, even within one category, some patients are more severely ill than others, some have more complications, some respond to treatment better than others etc etc. Crucially therefore the task is to identify groupings which make both medical sense – in that all patients in that group are clinically similar – and accounting sense – in that the treatment of all such patients will require similar resources. Although cumbersome, the expression 'resource homogeneous diagnosis related groups' well illustrates the problem. However, there is no reason to believe that it is incapable of solution. Probably it will require more categories of patients, coupled with some form of severity ratings. Nevertheless there are examples in the industrial/commercial world of organisations with several thousands of product variants. With modern data processing facilities the numbers of categories are not likely to be a problem.

Once we have definable categories of patients, each of which can have a defined treatment regime, it then becomes a fairly straightforward task to build up a defined treatment cost. Such an exercise involves setting standard costs for hospital units such as 'bed/days' and 'operating theatre hours' etc. This information can now readily be produced within existing clinical budgeting systems. In management accounting terms this is simply a standard product cost. Most industrial/commercial concerns will have such standard costs calculated for their ranges of products. They would regard them as essential information necessary to plan their activities, to prepare operating budgets and to assist in pricing their products.

All of the developments described above are concerned with the running costs, or 'revenue' expenditure in the NHS. Similar developments are in hand in respect of the *capital* expenditure. Before the reforms the NHS was much criticised because it did not have a comprehensive inventory of its fixed assets. It did not therefore have a commercial-type balance sheet which shows the value of those assets, nor did it take a 'depreciation' or 'leasing' charge for the use of those assets into its income and expenditure account.

However as with revenue expenditure, recognition of these weaknesses is not new. They too were identified in the Royal Commission and, similarly, there has been a series of developments in the intervening decade. Three are particularly significant.

First we have had the introduction in 1981 (DHSS 1981) of a more formal and comprehensive Investment Appraisal Mechanism known as the Appraisal of Options Procedure. This has since been refined with the issue of the revised Capricode (DHSS 1986) manual in 1986. Second we had the Ceri Davies Report of 1983 advocating the need for Health Authorities to develop an estate management plan. Third we had the 1985 Report by the then Association of Health Service Treasurers on Managing Capital Assets in the NHS (AHST 1985), in the light of which work was commissioned at three DHAs on setting up comprehensive asset systems.

Now no-one could argue that all the problems of financial management – particularly as an aid to achieving the maximum VFM from limited resources – had been overcome in the NHS. Indeed the opposite is the case. Across the whole of the NHS there had barely been a scratching of the surface. However all of the developments underway at the end of 1988 – involving both capital and revenue expenditure – shared three particular characteristics: they were evolutionary, they were ongoing and they were incomplete.

They were *evolutionary* in that, although many of the 'trials', 'pilot studies' and 'demonstrations' had different origins, there was frequently a common thread linking one to another, and lessons learned from one have been applied in another. They were *ongoing* in that they were still at an early stage and the process of applying them right across the whole of the NHS would take several years – probably up to the end of the century. Finally they were *incomplete* in that even on the pilot sites, many issues had yet to be addressed. Four in particular can readily be identified:

1 In the case of the RMI there is a need to coordinate activities in the acute hospitals with activities in community units and in family practitioner services to ensure – overall – the best VFM.

2 There is a need to introduce more comprehensive variance analysis to explain differences between 'budgeted' and 'actual' expenditure.

3 There is a need to tie together developments in revenue accounting with developments in capital and asset accounting to ensure that the impact of capital is properly accounted for.

4 There is a need to develop *flexible* budgeting to ensure that actual expenditure is measured against a budget which has been flexed to take account of *actual* workload (recognising both volume and mix factors). Flexible budgeting is normal practice in the industrial/commercial environment. In the context of acute hospitals in the NHS it is the logical next stage to follow case mix accounting, and could have been introduced with some changes to the 'old' funding structures of the NHS. The case for flexible budgets has been extensively argued by this writer elsewhere (Cook 1988). Several advantages can be identified, perhaps the most important of which is that it would remove the financial disincentive which existed for doctors, hospitals and Health Authorities to treat more patients.

Clearly then, at the end of 1988, there was a full and ongoing agenda for financial management within the NHS. Equally clearly it would have considerable implications for the staffing and structure of finance departments.

However that agenda did have the advantage that it could be developed on an evolutionary basis, and that further innovations could be incorporated without major upheaval.

Figure 3.4 shows the main elements of the then evolving structure of typical NHS finances functions deployed between RHAs, DHAs, Units and FPCs. Those elements already in place are shown in roman type. The Resource Management Initiative – which impacts primarily at Unit level – is shown in italics. Finally we can add these further developments which could reasonably have been anticipated. They are shown underlined.

Certainly there was a need for a substantial input of additional resources and the NHS needed to be more successful in attracting key staff such as accountants and computer staff. However there is a

RHAs:
Resource allocation
Financial planning
Capital expenditure control
Departmental budgeting
Payroll
Purchase accounts
Regional computer
Audit

FPCs:
Payments to contractors
Departmental budgeting
Payroll
F.P.S. Management Accounting

DHAs:
Financial planning
Departmental budgeting
Payroll
Purchase accounts
Income collection
Audit
Asset registers

Units
Departmental budgeting
Hospital information systems
Resource management
Developments of the RMI

Key
Normal Type – Present finance department components
Italics   – The resource management initiative
Underline   – Further developments

Figure 3.4   Typical pre-1991 NHS Finance Department structures, current and evolving

logical progression from present finance functions through to further developments. It is in this context that we need to assess the NHS reforms.

The NHS reforms

The *Working for Patients* White Paper created a new agenda.

There is one big financial feature which is unchanged. That is that 'the NHS is, and will continue to be, open to all, regardless of income, and financed mainly out of general taxation'. That, of course, is crucial. However there are many other changes within the reforms which clearly do impact on the financial structure and the need for better financial information and management. Indeed paragraph 1.17 of the White Paper listed five important aims of the changes, four of which were financial, namely:

1 To improve the information available to local managers, enabling them in turn to make their budgeting and monitoring more accurate, sensitive and timely.

2 To ensure that hospital consultants – whose decisions effectively commit sums of money – are involved in the management of hospitals; are given responsibility for the use of resources; and are encouraged to use those resources more effectively.

3 To contract out more functions which do not have to be undertaken by health authority staff and which could be provided more cost effectively by the private sector.

4 To ensure that drug prescribing costs are kept within reasonable limits.

Amongst the specific changes impacting on the finance function are:

1 The separation of responsibility for purchasing health care from that of providing health care. RHAs and DHAs now have planning commissioning and monitoring roles, while as many operational roles as possible are delegated to the hospitals.

2 Hospitals are able to apply for self governing status within the NHS as Hospital Trusts. They are not then funded directly but earn revenue from the services they provide.

3 NHS Hospital Trusts will be run by a Board of Directors – including a Director of Finance – on 'business-like' lines. They will therefore be free to retain surpluses and build up reserves, or to manage temporary deficits.

4 NHS Trusts will produce annual accounts which are similar in format to 'Companies Act' accounts. They therefore include a full balance sheet and income and expenditure account.
The liabilities side of the balance sheet includes:

(a) interest bearing debt, in respect of which interest payments must be made to the Department of Health;

(b) public dividend capital on which, in due course, dividends will be paid to the Treasury.

5 The assets of those hospitals becoming Trusts are vested in the Trust. Hence the Trust will manage its own capital programme and will be able to dispose of assets as it thinks appropriate and has borrowing powers, subject to an overall financing limit.

6 NHS Hospital Trusts can negotiate the pay and conditions of their own staff, and acquire their own supplies and services locally.

7 Contracts need to be negotiated between purchasers and providers for hospital services. These contracts will need to specify services supplied and prices can be in three forms:

(a) 'block' contracts for certain essential 'core' services;

(b) 'cost and volume' contracts specifying a price for a minimum level of service, with additional cases treated over that minimum to be supplied at agreed prices;

(c) 'cost per case' contracts.

8 A new system of resource allocation is replacing RAWP enabling money required to treat patients to be able to cross administrative boundaries.

9 A system of 'capital charges' is being introduced to reflect Health Authorities' use of existing capital assets and any new capital investment. The charges are set to cover the costs of interest and depreciation.

10 Family Health Services Authorities (successors to the Family Practitioner Committees) became accountable to RHAs and receive their funding from them.

11 Large GP practices are able to apply for their own practice budgets to enable them to purchase a defined range of services direct from hospitals.

12 There will be a closer monitoring of FHS drug expenditure. RHAs will distribute funds to FHSAs on a 'RAWP-like' weighted capitation formula. FHSAs will in turn monitor expenditure through 'Indicative Prescribing Amounts' for GP practices.

13 FHSAs, to continue the development towards actively managing – as opposed to purely administering – the FHS.

This is a formidable new agenda to be imposed – and implemented within a very short timescale – on top of the existing programme.

Space does not permit a detailed examination of each of these proposals. However within this chapter I do intend to comment on four aspects: First, there is the need to consider how the White Paper's proposals impact on the funding structure of the NHS. Second, there is the need to consider the consequent impact on finance departments. Third, some proposals do warrant a more detailed examination with regard to their desirability and practicability. In particular I wish to make some brief comments on five issues:

1 information for 'costs' and 'pricing';

2 the financial regime of NHS Trusts;

3 capital charges;

4 GP fundholding;

5 indicative prescribing.

Finally, I will draw some overall conclusions on the White Paper.

The funding structure

Figure 3.5 shows the funding structure of the NHS in England after the implementation of the reforms.

Clearly it shows a very much more complex structure that existed previously (Figure 3.1a). In fact the top half of the figure is not very different. The basic funding continues to come from the general taxation pool, supplemented by some income drawn from National Insurance contributions and some direct charges. The most significant change therefore in the top half is that funds for the Family Health Services now pass through the Regional Health Authorities, before being distributed to the Family Health Services Authorities. Figure 3.5 therefore requires a different layout from Figure 3.1a, with the RHAs centre stage and DHAs beneath them on the left and FHSAs on the right. There is however one further difference affecting the top half of the diagram. That is that the interest payments that NHS Hospital Trusts make go back to the NHS Management Executive. They in turn must then be distributed back into the system (to ensure that the overall level of funding provided by the Government is unchanged). Hence the amount provided for the Hospital and Community Health Services revenue must be supplemented by the amount of the NHS Hospital Trusts' interest payments. The interest payments are shown as the —·— lines in Figure 3.5.

It is in the bottom half of the figure that the dramatic changes occur. First, on the bottom line of the figure it is necessary to add three additional 'boxes': one for NHS Hospital Trusts, one for fundholding GPs (FHGPs), and one for private hospitals. We can then show the direct payments (--- lines) which are similar to those which are currently made although, there are some differences. We have already noted that FHSAs are to receive their funds from RHAs, there will also be payments for practice budgets from RHAs to FHGPs. They, however, will continue to receive some payments from their FHSAs.

Second, we need to add the capital charges. These are represented by the —— lines. The intention here is that they should operate down to individual budget holders. Accordingly we need to show capital charges returning from DMUs, back through DHAs to RHAs. As with interest charges, these then have to be redistributed. Hence the distribution of HCHS revenue funds from RHAs and DHAs and to FHGPs needs to be enhanced by the capital charges element.

Third, we need to consider the indicative prescribing amounts being introduced to control GP drug prescribing costs. The actual payment to pharmacists continues to be made as previously. Indicative prescribing acts as an aid to monitoring the prescribing costs of GPs rather than as a direct cash payment to them from which they pay the pharmacists. They therefore flow down from the FHSAs to the (non-fundholding) GPs with the actual expenditure incurred flowing in the opposite direction.

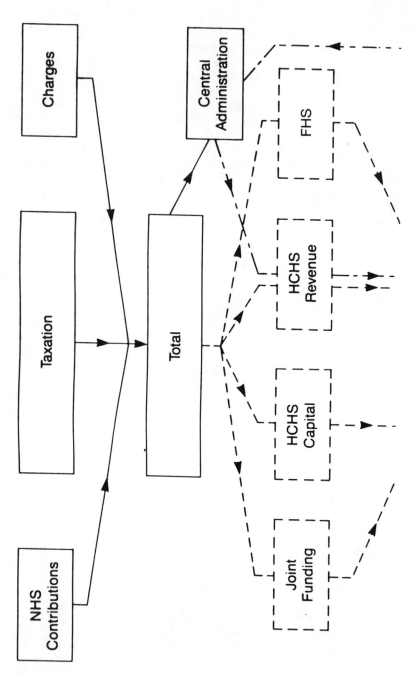

Figure 3.5   NHS funding in England post- *Working for Patients*

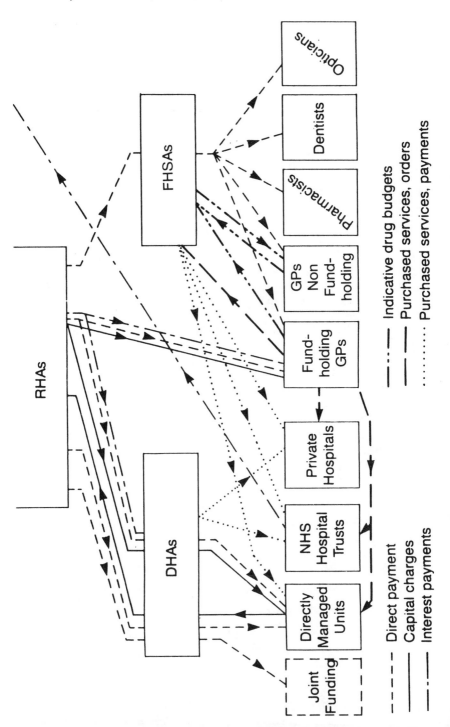

In the case of FHGPs the drugs element is included within the 'fund'. However the practice remains accountable to the FHSA for its drugs expenditure. In this case, therefore, there is one line running back from FHGPs to the FHSAs. The indicative prescribing amounts are the –· ·– lines in Figure 3.5.

Finally, we need to add the purchased services. These are shown as the ..... lines in the figure. The intention is that DHAs will purchase some of their services (under the three alternative forms of contract) from NHS Hospital Trusts and from private hospitals. Similarly FHGPs will purchase certain types of hospital treatment from NHS Hospital Trusts, DMUs and from some private hospitals. However they will simply place the orders, the cash will flow from the FHSAs. Thus in the figure we have the placing of orders shown as — — lines, while the actual flow of cash is shown as a .... line.

The impact on finance departments

Clearly this is a very different funding structure from that which existed previously and which is illustrated in Figure 3.1a. The first point we must consider then is simply the mechanics of making it work. Existing finance departments were not designed to handle this funding structure. Consequently there needs to be a massive overhaul. It will be an immense task and will take several years. It has been considered by groups within the Healthcare Financial Management Association (Webb 1989), and at some length by Prowle, Jones and Shaw (1989). Consequently I do not propose here to go into the impact on finance departments in detail. I have however illustrated the main sections which will need to exist – 'post reforms' – in Figure 3.6. It is involving a substantial input of accounting (and, of course, data processing) resources particularly where they did not exist previously: in directly managed hospitals, in NHS Hospital Trusts, in the FHSAs, and in the GP practices. Two years into the reform and the process has only just begun.

What is regrettable about this requirement is that it is for largely *financial* accounting facilities to address such issues as:

- How do we collect the income which is due to us?
- How do we pay for clinical services which we are purchasing?
- How do we pay for the goods and services which we need?
- How do we pay the wages?

It is in fact a diversion of resources *away* from the priorities which existed at the end of 1988 which were to develop the *management* accounting skills of the NHS: particularly to promote the better use of resources through the Resource Management Initiative.

Thus despite the fact that the reforms will require a substantial input of accounting resources these will be largely committed to

RHAs:	DHAs:	NHS Hospital trusts:
Resource allocation	Financial planning	Financial planning
Financial planning	Departmental	Departmental budgeting
Capital expenditure control	budgeting	Hospital information
Asset registers	Payroll	systems
Capital charges	Purchase accounts	Resource management
Departmental budgeting	Income collection	systems
Payroll	Asset registers	Payroll
Purchase accounts	Capital charges	Purchase accounts
Regional computer	Audit	Sales accounts
Audit		Capital expenditure
		control
DMUs:	**FPCs:**	Asset registers
Financial planning	Payments to contractors	Interest payments
Departmental budgeting	Departmental budgeting	Audit
Hospital information	Payroll	
systems	Indicative drug budgets	**GP Practices:**
Resource management	G.P. Practice budgets	Indicative drug budgets
systems	F.P.S. management	Practice budgets. (Where
Payroll	accounting	appropriate)
Purchase accounts	Audit	
Sales accounts		
Asset registers		
Capital charges		
Audit		

Figure 3.6   Typical NHS finance deparment structures post-'Working for patients'

the bureaucratic tasks of coordinating transactions between A and B. Already surveys within the Healthcare Financial Management Association suggest that between 1.8 and 2.0 per cent of HCHS revenue funding is committed to the *purchasing* function. If we assume that a similar amount is committed to the *sales* function then up to 4 per cent of revenue resources are being applied simply to the mechanisms of operating the market. Currently that is some £600 million per annum. Given particularly the Governments' record in the early 1980s of denouncing the 'excessive' administrative costs of the NHS that seems incredible.

Some specific proposals considered

Pricing, costing and the Resource Management Initiative
A fragmented NHS, in which various organisations buy and sell clinical services from one another on a 'businesslike' basis, requires information for pricing. The White Paper made the bland assumption that this would be provided by the Resource Management Initiative.

There are two major misconceptions here. First there is the issue of the timetable for 'rolling out' the RMI to the 260 major acute units. WFP also made the statement that the RMI would be 'extended and accelerated' with the aim of building up coverage to those units by the end of 1991/2, ie March 1992. There was never any prospect of that happening and, of course, it has not happened. Now one year further on the number of RM sites which can provide any meaningful case-mix costs can be counted on the fingers of one hand. My view has always been, and still is, that the extension of the RMI will still be with us in the year 2000.

A more serious misconception is that the RMI is designed to provide the appropriate information for pricing. This was never the intention of the RMI. As we have already discussed in this chapter, the case-mix accountancy developments within the RMI are still in their infancy. The six pilot sites are concentrating on the use of DRGs (and their successors HRGs) which cover only adult acute inpatients. Outpatients (and other categories) are not covered. In addition there is much evidence that DRG/HRGs are not the appropriate classifications for pricing purposes even within adult acute inpatient cases. Certainly they do not correspond to the categories identified within WFPs, GP practice budgets. Prowle, Jones and Shaw (1989) suggest that Treatment Related Groups might be more appropriate. TRGs is a concept, first identified by Gambling (1987) in which patients are classified more according to the treatment they receive than according to their clinical classification.

What is clear, is that any newly appointed Director of Finance in an NHS Hospital Trust will be concerned about his inability to price his products. Thus once he has overcome his immediate problems of how to pay the wages he will then require the development of an internal standard costing and budgetary control system which does give him the information he requires.

In the only comprehensive survey to date of NHS costing Ellwood (1992) concludes: 'the role of the NHS accountant in ensuring the successful developments of the NHS internal market centres around his ability to deliver on costing and pricing contracts. Existing cost methods are far from adequate to ensure an efficient allocation of healthcare resources through the internal market'.

The financial regime of NHS Trusts
What is emerging from two years' experience of the reforms is that the NHS Trusts will not be quite the free-wheeling entrepreneurial organisations that the early expectations of their role suggested.

Certainly the financial regime is, in some respects, very different from that of a 'traditional' DHA. They are to produce annual accounts of a balance sheet, an income and expenditure account, and a source and application of funds statement that correspond as closely as possible to private sector, Companies Acts accounts. We have already discussed the new structures that are required for the finance departments.

However what is also emerging is the nature of financial constraints which are being imposed upon them. They are threefold:

1 to deliver a 6 per cent return on capital employment;

2 to balance their income and expenditure account (after taking the 6 per cent ROCE);

3 to live within their (annually negotiated) external funding limit.

These three constraints broadly operate on the balance sheet, the income and expenditure account, and the source and application of funds statement. Collectively they mean that the Trust has very little latitude and is committed to the business plans that it has agreed with the NHS Management Executive.

However reservations emerge in respect of whether these constraints are workable once the 'free-market' really does come into play. In particular how realistic is the requirement for a Trust to deliver 6 per cent ROCE? The early experience of some Trusts is that the Department of Health is not interested in a return of 5.9 per cent, nor is it interested in a return of 6.1 per cent. The requirement is for 6.0 per cent.

Now in the early days of the market, when most contracts are still 'block' contracts supplemented by a few 'cost and volume' contracts, with a little creative accounting, most Trusts will deliver 6.0 per cent. However once cost-per-case contracts become the norm, and the volume and mix of cases within a Trust's actual workload differ substantially from those budgeted, then Trusts are going to find it extremely difficult to hit a 6.0 per cent target ROCE. In fact it won't work.

Capital charges
A feature of the reforms was the introduction of a system of capital charges. They have three objectives:

1 to increase awareness in health service managers of the cost of capital;

2 to create incentives to use capital efficiently;

3 to see NHS provision evaluated on a basis broadly comparable with the private sector.

Note, however, that funds for NHS capital investment continue to be provided by the Exchequer as a separate allocation within the overall programme. Capital *charges* therefore impact the distribution of *revenue* funds to Health Authorities. Capital accounting is a difficult area and no one would seriously argue that previous NHS practice was satisfactory. Indeed the need for Health Authorities to hold comprehensive asset registers was no more than basic accounting.

However, the authors of the reforms have not thought the matter through and have come up with a set of proposals which will simply divert attention away from the real agenda which does exist for NHS capital accounting. Certainly it can be argued that the Government's objectives are not achieved.

First, capital charges based on *fixed assets* actually divert attention away from an area where NHS managers can make more efficient use of capital: that is in the control of *working capital*. Decisions affecting fixed assets are, by their nature, ad hoc and occasional. The control of working capital is an every day activity and managers *should* direct more attention say to stock levels of consumable items. Capital charges are useless in this context. Hence the proposals fail on their No. 1 objective.

Second, Working Paper 5 of WFP stated that 'Authorities will need to keep asset registers and calculate capital charges for each functional unit so that budgetary and costing systems also reflect managerial responsibility for assets'. This implies that capital charges will go right down to the departmental level in the budgetary control system. Now in the private sector not all companies take depreciation into their management accounts. There is a very sound reason for this in that depreciation is not a cash item and is one over which the departmental manager has little control. Let us assume, for example, that a budget is agreed for a department and includes depreciation (or capital charges) of £12,000 for the year.

After month 1 the operating statement reads:
    Depreciation: Budget £1000, Actual £1000
After month 2 it reads:
    Depreciation: Budget £1000, Actual £1000
Month 3 likewise:
    Depreciation: Budget £1000, Actual £1000

By now the item is beginning to lose its impact and by month 6 it will have no significance whatsoever. Moreover the incentive to the department manager will completely disappear when he/she realises that there is no virement: thus even if he can reduce his capital charge by £500 per month, this will not give him an extra £300 to spend on other items. Thus objective No. 2 has not been achieved.

Third the capital charges are to include 'depreciation' and an 'interest' element. That of course is not comparable to the private sector where the return on capital element falls in the margin between calculated 'costs' and selling prices. In addition assets are to be revalued (now) at intervals of 5 years. However, this too is not private sector practice. The private sector has, in fact, been struggling with the intricacies of inflation accounting for the last 25 years and has, by and large, abandoned the idea as being too difficult. Certainly there is no requirement in private hospitals to revalue their fixed assets every 5 years. Hence far from seeing NHS provision evaluated on a basis broadly comparable with the private sector, the authors of WFP have swung the balance in favour of private hospitals. Objective No. 3 is not achieved.

Finally, there is the issue of how precisely capital charges will impact on the funds that DHAs actually receive. Working Paper 9 of WFP purported to show this but was sadly, incomprehensible. It did not give an example of how revenue expenditure is allocated down to Regions, Districts and Units, and the 'before and after' cases of their allocations showing the impact of capital charges, and how they will change when

Districts or Units actually increase or decrease their employment of fixed assets.

Two years into the reforms the mechanisms for capital charges and resource allocation remain confused.

In fact with regard to fixed assets there are two important requirements to ensure that they are deployed efficiently. First there is the need to get the original *investment appraisal* right. Here the NHS has made considerable progress in recent years since the introduction of the Appraisal of Options procedure. Second, there is the need to create a funding structure whereby managers are encouraged to treat as many patients are possible. If they can do that they will be using their resources (including fixed assets) efficiently. Flexed budgets coupled with case-mix accounting promises that.

Thus while there is a major agenda for capital accounting in the NHS, the reforms do not provide the solution.

Fundholding GP practices
It is perhaps the Family Health Services which offer the biggest challenge to those seeking to promote better value for money. The reforms made a number of structural and organisational changes – including the appointment of FHSA General Managers – which are to be welcomed. They may be seen as steps in the transition from the Family Health Services being purely 'administered' services to being pro-actively managed

To the management accountant the challenge offered by the FHS is tremendous. Previously the finance function within the FPCs had been largely a 'pay and rations' operation of paying to the doctors, dentists, pharmacists and opticians the allowances to which they are entitled in the 'Red Book' (DHSS 1979).

Now we have the prospect of organisations which must establish objectives, identify priorities within those objectives, allocate resources and then monitor expenditure against the achievement of those priorities and objectives. This within a total turnover in England of £6 billion. It is a very exciting challenge and one which is largely overdue. Sadly the fundholding proposals are a diversion from this. What they will do is give the GPs a role to play in allocating resources to the Hospital Services and will contribute nothing to the delivery of better VFM within the FHS. At best they will be a smoke screen diverting attention away from how the GPs deliver their services. At worst they will be a cumbersome and bureaucratic nightmare which involves sending patients to distant, low priced hospitals.

Indicative prescribing accounts
In contrast the proposals for indicative prescribing are not so much wrongly conceived as incomplete. GPs make many decisions which have financial consequences and all the arguments for clinical budgets

to be applied to hospital doctors can also be applied to GPs. Certainly, to the accountant there is no reason why those doctors who are high spenders in their prescribing habits should not be held to be financially accountable for their decisions. However GPs make many other decisions which have financial consequences. They ask for pathology tests to be conducted by the local hospitals, they call on the community health services, and they refer patients to hospital for inpatient treatment. Consequently it is correct to assess the standard of service being provided by a GP, against the resources he is committing.

However, there are dangers in examining their drug spending patterns in isolation – particularly where the express aim of the White Papers was 'to apply downward pressure on drug expenditure' – without assessing the other factors and whether such constraints really do deliver better VFM. As a first stage in developing better financial management in the FHS 'indicative prescribing' does have a role to play. However it is no more than a first stage.

Conclusions

In this chapter I have tried to assess the reforms in the light of the financial management agenda that existed at the end of 1988. I have endeavoured to look at the principles behind its proposals, rather than the detailed systems requirements necessary to make them work.

In diagrammatic form the reforms are changing the funding situation of the NHS from that shown in Figure 3.1a to that shown in Figure 3.5. Similarly the impact on the finance function will require a transition from Figure 3.4 to 3.3.

The White Paper placed great emphasis on the fact that currently 'hospitals which offer the best VFM are not rewarded for doing so. Indeed hospitals may be penalised for this efficiency if they succeed in treating more patients than they had budgeted for'. However that defect – which is considerable – can be overcome by introducing fixed budgets as an extension to the RMI. Therefore the only additional benefits which can be identified in Figure 3.5 are those which might accrue from the competitive structure which the Government is creating. Clearly the additional costs of such a structure are enormous. There is no evidence that the benefits from 'competition' outweigh the administrative cost involved. What is clear is that the system will only work if hospitals really do need to compete with one another to obtain their business. That means that there must be some slack in the system, and the Government will ensure that this is so by continuing to cash limit the NHS in total. It is therefore, by definition, setting out not to use all the NHS facilities to the greatest extent. As long as there is a waiting list for hospital treatment, that is not maximising VFM.

As a final thought let's recap on the introduction of resource management and the lessons which had to be learned from the earlier management budgeting experience. They were identified in HN (86)34:

1 Doctors and nurses need to be centrally involved in management arrangements.

2 Doctors and nurses need to be centrally involved in specifying information requirements.

3 Effective financial management support is vital.

4 The pace at which new financial systems can be introduced needs to be carefully judged.

These lessons are equally valid in respect of the NHS reforms and demonstrate that it will actually be several years before the success of the reforms can be assessed.

References

AHST 1985 *Managing Capital Assets in the NHS* AHST/CIPFA.

Blyth, J 1983 *Budgetary Control/Management Budgeting* Unpublished.

Cmd 249 1987 *Promoting Better Health: The Governments Programme for Improving Primary Health Care* HMSO.

Cook, AN (with Perrin, J) 1988 *Funding the NHS: Which Way Forward?* NAHA.

Cook, AN 1988 'Managing Britain's health services: Why the best option may yet lie within' *Financial Times* 16 March 1988.

DHSS 1979 *Statement of Fees and Allowances Payable to General Medical Practitioners in England and Wales* DHSS.

DHSS 1981 *Health Notice (81)30: Health Services Management. Health Building Procedures* DHSS.

DHSS 1983 *Underused and Surplus Property in the NHS: Report of the Enquiry* HMSO.

DHSS 1986 *Capricode: Health Building Procedures* HMSO.

DHSS 1986 *Health Notice (86)34: Resource Management (Management Budgeting) in Health Authorities* DHSS.

DHSS 1986 *The Health Service in England: Annual Report 1985–86* DHSS.

DHSS 1992 *NHS Annual Accounts 1990–91* HMSO.

Ellwood, S 1992 *Cost Methods for NHS Healthcare Contracts* CIMA.

Gambling T 1987 'Baumol's disease, group technology and the NHS' *Financial Accountability and Management* 3, 1, 47–58.

Maynard, A 1984 'Budgeting in health care systems' *Effective Health Care* 2, 2, 41–48.

NHS/DHSS 1984 *Steering Group on Health Services Information: Sixth Report to the Secretary of State* HMSO.

Prowle, M, Jones, T and Shaw J, 1989 *Working for Patients: The Management of Financial Resources in the NHS* HMSO.

Royal Commission on the NHS 1978 *Research Paper No. 2 Management of Financial Resources in the NHS* HMSO.

Webb, N 1989 'Taking the NHS finance function into the 1990s' *Public Finance and Accountancy* 10 November 1989.

4 Assessing efficiency in the new NHS

Mike Drummond

Introduction

Increased efficiency is one of the major objectives of the White Paper *Working for Patients* (DoH 1989a). The document proposes a number of efficiency promoting measures, including the establishment of an 'internal market' for health services with contracts between 'purchasers' and 'providers', a voluntary scheme for those general practices that wish to manage their own budget and indicative drug budgets for all general practitioners.

Since the pursuit of increased efficiency is one of the major objectives of the proposals, this begs the question of how efficiency will be assessed. Chapter 2 in this volume (Mullen) points out that the functioning of the internal market in health care is not a simple matter. One cannot necessarily assume that the operation of market principles *per se* will automatically lead to efficiency. Indeed, there is considerable evidence from the literature (Evans 1985) that this is *not* the case, whether the patient is the direct consumer of services, or whether the doctor acts as an agent on the patient's behalf.

There has been relatively little formal assessment of the efficiency of alternative health care programmes or treatments in the United Kingdom (Ludbrook and Mooney 1983, Drummond and Hutton 1987). Authors point to a number of possible explanations including the lack of appropriate evaluative skills, the lack of available data and the lack of appropriate incentives. Indeed, the only formal requirement for economic evaluation of alternative plans or programmes at the current time is that of *option appraisal* for schemes where one of the options is a capital scheme with an initial outlay of £10 million or more (DHSS 1981). In such cases, the Regional Health Authority needs to submit a formal evaluation of the costs and benefits of options with its approval in principle submission to the Department of Health (Akehurst 1989).

In addition, the Department of Health undertakes, or commissions, evaluations of health technologies at the national level (Buxton *et al.*

1985) and has issued guidance on the economic evaluation of medical equipment (DHSS 1988). However, it has neither been thought desirable nor feasible to require formal evaluations of alternative programmes, treatments or technologies at the local level. Rather, the emphasis has been on reviewing Health Authority performance on a more aggregate level, through the development of performance indicators (DHSS 1983), supported by the review process. There is no equivalent exhaustive review of family practitioner services, which are a major focus of the recent White Paper and the subject of an additional White Paper on primary health care (DoH 1989b).

This chapter examines the prospects and problems of assessing the efficiency of health care alternatives in the light of the recent White Paper.; In particular, it considers the following issues:

(a) what methods are available for assessing the efficiency of health care programmes and treatments;

(b) in what ways are the White Paper proposals likely to encourage assessment of efficiency;

(c) what monitoring systems should be put in place to assess whether more efficient health care provision has been secured as a result of the White Paper?

Methods for assessing the efficiency of health care programmes

The methods of economic evaluation have been well documented elsewhere so will only briefly be described here (Drummond 1980, Warner and Luce 1982, Drummond *et al.* 1987). There are several related techniques, all having the common feature that some combination of the inputs (resources consumed) by health care programmes are compared with some combination of the outputs (improvements in health obtained).

The particular techniques differ mainly in the extent to which they measure and value improvements in health. Some techniques, such as *cost analysis* and *cost minimisation analysis*, proceed on the basis that the alternatives under consideration have been shown to be equivalent in effectiveness. Others, such as *cost–utility analysis* and *cost–benefit analysis*, measure health improvements in quality-adjusted life-years and money terms respectively. The most widely used technique is *cost–effectiveness analysis*, where the costs are measured in money terms and the improvements in health assessed in the most convenient natural units, such as 'years of life gained' or 'disability days avoided'. (The various forms of analysis are outlined in Figure 4.1).

There are two features of economic evaluation that merit particular emphasis in the light of the White Paper proposals. First, assessment of efficiency *explicitly* requires consideration of *both* the resource use

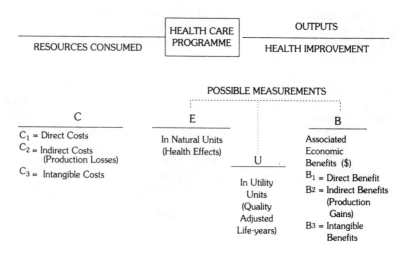

Figure 4.1 Components of economic evaluation

and the improvements in health obtained from the use of health care interventions. Therefore, improvements in efficiency need to be distinguished from cost-cutting measures, where no consideration is given to the reduction in the effectiveness of the programme when the resource commitment is reduced. Therefore, in the context of contracts for clinical services, or the establishment of community drugs formularies, the lowest cost option is not necessarily the most efficient.

Second, assessment of efficiency implies a *wide* consideration of the costs of health care programmes. For example, the consideration of cost is not restricted to the hospital, but includes also the costs in primary care and those borne by patients and their families. In the past, there has been a tendency in the NHS to shift costs from Health Authority to family practitioner committee budgets, through the earlier discharge of patients from hospital, or through restrictions in drug prescribing on hospital discharge. (Conversely, long waiting times for an outpatient attendance or for hospital admission also shift costs from secondary care to primary care. In the average district general hospital a significant proportion of medical admissions are emergencies.)

A key aspect of the White Paper proposals is the Health Authority and family practitioner budgets are more interrelated. At the level of the Regional Health Authority, they are combined. In addition, those general practices wishing to administer their own budgets have included in their budgets a component to cover certain hospital-based treatments. However, this falls short of the health maintenance organisation (HMO) concept in the USA, where all the health care of enrollees is a charge on the HMO (Drummond and Maynard 1988). Nevertheless, the White Paper proposals should, in principle, change the behaviour of key actors, such as general practitioners, in respect of the costs they consider relevant to their decisions.

Impact of the White Paper proposals on the assessment of efficiency

It was mentioned earlier that, with the exception of option appraisal, the application of economic evaluation methods is limited in the NHS to date. In 1987, Drummond and Hutton undertook a review of the economic appraisal of health technology. They found that 50 economic appraisals had been published, covering a wide range of topics. This is still minute in relation to the number of health technologies used in the NHS, however.

It is possible that Drummond and Hutton's review underestimates the total activity, since many appraisals may be undertaken within health authorities and such reports do not always enter into the public domain. This could be the case, but there is no evidence to suggest that the amount of 'in-house' appraisal is extensive. Indeed, in situations where Health Authorities have had easy access to the skills of economists, as through the York Health Economics Consortium (University of York, 1990), demand has been high, suggesting that the appropriate skills for the assessment of efficiency have been lacking in the past.

It is much more likely that the majority of assessments are currently undertaken either informally or indirectly. For example, the managers in most authorities trust their clinical staff to be applying the most appropriate treatment technologies, either in their day-to-day practice, or in submitting bids for the development of clinical services. The extent to which this trust is misplaced is unknown. Managers mainly comfort themselves in the knowledge that physical and financial resources for clinical work are in short supply in the NHS. This is therefore likely to encourage clinicians to search for most cost-effective procedures. However, it is known from the research into performance indicators that clinical teams with similar levels of resources produce different amounts of services (Yates and Davidge 1984). Also it is conceivable that cash limits, whilst being effective in capping overall expenditure, may militate against the adoption of new, cost-effective, procedures if these necessitate financial outlays.

The discussion above has related mainly to the services under the management of Health Authorities. Even less is known about the assessment of efficiency in family practitioner services. General practitioners are largely free to employ the treatment technologies, mainly pharmaceuticals, that they see fit, with no overall budgetary limitation. Similarly, there are no restrictions on referrals to secondary care, although long waiting times act as a limitation in practice.

Given the current arrangements in primary and secondary care, it is hardly surprising that there has been so little assessment of efficiency to date. There is little or no formal requirement and few incentives. As the White Paper proposals are implemented, the incentives have changed quite considerably. The next sections of this chapter examine a number of the key proposals in relation to the impact they may have on the assessment of efficiency.

The internal market in health care

For the first time, an element of competition has been injected into the provision of health care through the NHS. District Health Authorities, through their role as purchasers, enter into contracts with a number of agencies, including their own directly managed units, to secure health services on behalf of their population. The extent of choice available to the DHA purchasers will vary from one location to another, but is being broadened through the advent of self-governing NHS Trusts and the existence of a number of private hospitals.

The providers, be they directly NHS managed or self-governing, are not guaranteed a budget as in the past. Rather they attract funds as a direct result of the contracts placed. In addition to the contracts placed by Health Authorities, others will come from those general practitioners who opt to manage their own budget.

The precise extent to which competitive forces will come into play is as yet uncertain. One current concern of district general managers is the apparent paradox between, on the one hand, the need to secure good value for money in health care for the population served and, on the other hand, the need to ensure that one's own directly managed units do not fail (Crump *et al.* 1990). The view taken by the district on the relative importance of these two needs is likely to be a large influence on the competitive pressures faced by a given unit, as is the existence locally of other public or private providers and the number of GP budget-holders.

However, although the extent of competition will vary from place to place, all providers need to begin thinking about their business plan. Namely, what markets are they seeking to serve and how are they going to serve them. Since the price at which services are marketed will also be a factor, one would expect that the business planning exercise will prompt an examination of the treatment technologies being employed and their relative cost-effectiveness. Some providers have already gone as far as to produce prospectuses outlining their services. Though these documents do not necessarily show evidence of cost-effectiveness thinking being employed in their production, they are the first sign that market forces are having an impact.

Contracts for clinical services

The White Paper working paper on funding and contracts for hospital services envisages three broad classes of contract; *block contracts*, under which the GP or DHA would pay the hospital an annual fee in return for access to a defined range of services; *cost and volume contracts*, under which hospitals would receive a sum in respect of a baseline level of activity, defined in terms of a given number of treatments or cases, and *cost per case contracts*, where payment would be made to the hospital on a case by case basis, without any prior commitment of either party to the volume of cases which might be so dealt with.

Although the precise management arrangements for each type of contract will differ, the contracting procedure will incorporate several key steps, many of which offer the opportunity for assessment of efficiency. In particular, someone, maybe the DHA or the individual GP, needs to decide whether contracts are to be let for particular services or not. Once this has been decided, a contract specification needs to be written outlining the services to be provided, the treatment technologies to be used, the volume of cases to be treated, the standards to be achieved (in clinical effectiveness and quality of care) and price. Finally, a monitoring system needs to be put in place to see that the work specified in the contract has been undertaken to the required standard within the agreed financial amount. Any deviations from the terms and conditions of the contract would thus have to be justified. These decision points are discussed in turn below.

Deciding whether or not to place a contract
In reality, the scope for choice here will depend on the nature of the clinical service concerned and the room for political manoeuvre. For example, the provision of emergency services locally may not be a matter of choice, although there are, no doubt, choices relating to the nature and extent of emergency cover, eg number of accident and emergency units in a given geographical area and the extent of 24 hours a day, 7 days a week cover. For certain types of elective operation, there is likely to be much more scope for choice in whether or not to let contracts.

There is scope here for economic evaluation to inform priorities for health care. For example, Williams (1985) pointed out that coronary artery bypass grafting for severe angina with left main disease gave much better value for money (£1,040 per Quality-Adjusted Life-Year (QALY) gained in 1983–84 prices) than CABG for mild angina with two vessel disease (£12,600 per QALY gained).

Under the current arrangements, the priorities within open heart surgery are decided solely by the clinicians concerned. The DHA merely decides the level at which it is prepared to fund its surgical unit. One would expect that, all things being equal, clinical priorities would determine that the most serious cases are operated upon first, with broader and broader indications being accepted as funding becomes more widely available. However, this is not currently an *explicit* agreement between management and the clinical staff. Indeed, it is possible that clinicians would treat cases which they find particularly interesting or challenging from a clinical viewpoint, rather than those which offer the most returns (in terms of health improvement) in relation to the cost. Many surgical waiting lists comprise large numbers of simple, low cost, procedures. For example, an analysis of ophthalmology waiting lists has shown that the vast majority of patients are waiting for cataract extraction (Drummond and Yates 1988). However, crude calculations of the cost per QALY gained from cataract extraction show this to be a high value for money procedure (Drummond 1988). A similar situation exists in orthopaedics, where hip replacement has been demonstrated to give good value for money (Williams 1985).

Under the new arrangements, DHAs and GPs will be able to decide which clinical needs should be met first through their ability to place contracts. In that respect, the White Paper represents a major shift in decision-making about health care priorities. The extent to which DHAs and GPs will exercise their new power remains to be seen, although the waiting list initiative (IACC 1989) demonstrates that the letting of contracts with units, or the threat of taking the funds elsewhere, has led to change in behaviour of secondary care physicians.

However, one benefit for DHAs and GPs of the present system is that difficult rationing decisions are taken by hospital physicians and are seldom made explicit. In that respect, physicians take on an additional burden beyond their immediate remit. It may be that DHAs, in particular, will find the explicitness that accompanies the placing of contracts difficult to contend with. It will now be their responsibility to explain to the public why some cases are priorities and others not. Economic evaluation and the calculation of comparative costs per quality-adjusted life-year gained is one way of providing such an explanation. It remains to be seen whether Health Authorities will take tough decisions and then seek to justify them, or whether they will seek ways to preserve the existing system, where rationing decisions are not made explicit. In practice, this would lead DHAs to opt more for block contracts, or cost and volume contracts with very flexible arrangements for overruns.

Deciding upon the contract specification
Under the current arrangements, the hospital physicians largely decide on the method of treatment and (implicitly) the cost. It has been pointed out (Akehurst and Drummond 1989) that, while managers take some of the decisions controlling resource allocation, such as the nature of the 'hotel' facilities in hospitals, the major resource allocators are the doctors. They decide when to admit the patient, the nature of the diagnostic workup, the treatment technologies to be employed and when to discharge.

With the advent of contracts, a specification for the care to be provided will be drawn up. The level of detail in this specification is currently not clear, and there are at present very few examples of contracts (Drummond, Marchment and Crump 1989, Central Birmingham Health Authority 1989, Department of Health 1990). Drummond *et al.* (1989) argue that it is important to specify contracts in considerable detail, including the client group to be served, the treatment methods to be applied, the standards of care to be achieved and the arrangements for monitoring.

Since a key feature of the contract will be the stated price, this gives an excellent opportunity for comparisons of options. For example, different treatment technologies may have different cost-effectiveness. Taking a simple case, there may be evidence that day-care or short-stay surgery is just as effective, but of lower cost, then traditional surgery (Russell *et al.* 1977, Waller *et al.* 1978). Therefore providers ought to be able to agree to contracts for these services at a lower price. Costs may also vary with volume. Although this has been relatively under explored by economists (Labelle 1987), presumably those providers concentrating on certain clinical services may be able to agree large contracts at a lower implied unit price. An example of this would be the concerted efforts to clear the cataract backlog (Thomas *et al.* 1989).

Finally, there may be occasions where there is an explicit trade-off between higher costs and higher quality. This may be in terms of amenities in hospital wards, or in the actual clinical care provided. For example, some surgical implants may have a greater durability or offer greater freedom of movement to the patient than others. In cataract surgery, a posterior changer intraocular lens offers a greater quality of eyesight than aphakic spectacles (Davies *et al.* 1986). Here, part of the contracting process will be for the purchaser to make explicit decisions about the level of quality required. In essence, this requires assessment of whether the extra benefits exceed the higher costs. Providers may decide to offer a range of options at differing price.

Economic evaluation, with its explicit assessment of costs and health improvement, is again well placed to offer essential data to inform these choices. In the past they have been made implicitly by the providers, although general practitioners may have adjusted their referral patterns based on knowledge about their patients' preferences and clinical practice in given hospitals. Such 'consumer choice' exercised through the GP, has probably been most prominent in the field of maternity care to date.

One concern is whether competition in health care will drive out quality. The evidence on this, mainly from the USA, is mixed (Drummond 1990). However, if economic evaluation were used more frequently in choosing between treatment technologies such 'trade-offs' between cost and quality would be made more explicit. Also, economic evaluation would ensure that an appropriate *range* of costs is considered when cost comparisons are being made.

Deciding upon contract monitoring arrangements

Although an important feature of the contracting procedure, this is one where economic evaluation currently has little to offer. Most evaluations of health technologies are performed *ex ante* and there are few examples of situations where researchers have investigated whether the preferred option as indicated by their study has performed well in practice.

However, it is clear that the monitoring of contracts is not a costless exercise and it is known from more aggregate economic studies that the administrative costs of health care systems embodying a significant market element are much higher than those of the NHS (Maxwell 1985). Therefore, there is a role for the economic evaluation of alternative monitoring arrangements; namely, does the increased cost of more comprehensive monitoring generate benefits in the closer adherence to contract specifications?

Practice budgets for general medical practitioners

Under the terms of the White Paper, practices serving at least 11,000 patients will be able to manage their own budget. (Under certain circumstances the DH have indicated that this limit could be dropped to 9,000.) The budget will cover various hospital services (such as a defined group of surgical inpatient and day-case treatment covering most elective procedures, outpatient services and diagnostic investigation of patients and specimens) and practice services and prescribing.

In general concept, the practice budget scheme is similar to that of the Health Maintenance Organisation (HMO) in the United States. Whilst not nearly as extensive, it embodies several of the same incentives, such as to improve the range and quality of one's own services in order to attract more patients and to review carefully the appropriateness of utilising certain hospital services. Whereas the White Paper working paper dealing with this topic points out that 'the scheme will be structured to ensure that GPs have no financial incentives to refuse to treat any category of patients', it is well known that, in the USA, HMOs reduced the number of hospital admissions dramatically. They also made much greater use of other health care professionals, such as nurse practitioners (Drummond and Maynard 1988). Whether or not these changes, whilst reducing costs, also brought about a reduction in the quality of care is open to debate (Ware *et al.* 1986).

Much of what was said above about contracts for clinical services also applies to GPs operating their own budgets. They will have an interest in knowing that the treatment technologies used in the secondary care sector are the most cost-effective available. Additionally, GPs will be able to consider whether it is more cost-effective to refer patients to the hospital at all, or to handle the care themselves. An obvious issue would be the substitution of careful management by the GP ambulatory care, rather than requesting hospital admission. Also, some GPs already undertake minor elective surgery. Perhaps this will increase if it can be shown, in a cost minimisation analysis, to be equally effective but of lower cost.

Another major item of GP care is pharmaceutical consumption. This component of the practice budget allocated by Regions will be in accordance with the principles outlined for indicative budgets (discussed below). However, it may have extra meaning for GPs operating the practice budget scheme if increased expenditure on drugs means that other items of expenditure, such as elective admission to hospital, are reduced.

For example, it has recently been shown that a new drug (misoprostol), if used prophylactically, can reduce the incidence of non-steroidal anti-inflammatory drug (NSAID) associated ulcers in those patients taking these drugs for their arthritis (Graham *et al.* 1988). Should the GP prescribe the additional drug? This question could be answered by an economic evaluation of the prophylactic use of misoprostol. Similarly, prescribing long-term medication for elevated blood pressure or serum cholesterol will reduce the number of fatal and non-fatal coronary heart disease events. An economic evaluation could investigate the costs and benefits of such actions (Drummond and McGuire 1990).

Indicative prescribing budgets for general medical practitioners

The working paper dealing with this topic argues that 'it is generally recognised that some prescribing is wasteful or unnecessarily expensive. The objective of the new arrangements is to place downward pressure on expenditure on drugs in order to limit this waste and to release resources for other parts of the Health Service'.

Despite this forthright tone, later parts of the document point out that 'the scheme will be structured in a way that patients will always get the drugs they need' and that 'it will ensure that budgets reflect the costs of patients needing a greater volume of drugs or more expensive drugs . . .' 'so that there will be no disincentive to practices to accept such patients or to begin to prescribe expensive medicine to such patients, if there is a clinical need to do so'.

The development of indicative prescribing budgets needs to be considered alongside two other initiatives; the feedback of information on prescribing behaviour to GPs through PACT (prescribing analyses and cost) and the development of community formularies. Therefore, whereas prescribing budgets will inevitably be set in the aggregate, taking into account local social and epidemiologists factors, both PACT and formularies are much more likely to lead the GP to consider why a particular drug, and not an alternative including no drug, should be given in a particular instance.

Both PACT and formularies will give information to GPs on drug costs. This is to be welcomed. However, Drummond (1989) has pointed out that there are dangers in drawing up formularies in a too simplistic way, merely considering the comparative costs of the drugs themselves.

First, it is possible that a too narrow definition of comparative costs would be used. This should not only consider the costs of the drugs but the other medical care that is required. For example, a slightly cheaper drug may require a more expensive route of administration, require more frequent patient monitoring, or lead to more side-effects.

Second, it is possible that costs in the longer term may be ignored.

This is particularly true of drugs that are used prophylactically, such as lipid lowering agents. These may require additional costs *now*, but the costs of coronary heart disease occurring in the future may be reduced. (Although in an economic evaluation, costs occurring in the future have less weight, since they are *discounted* to present values. See Drummond (1980) for more discussion.)

Third, it is possible that differences in the effectiveness of drugs will be ignored in the quest for cost-cutting. It was mentioned earlier that one must distinguish between economic efficiency and cost-cutting. Therefore, it is conceivable that a higher cost drug would be worthwhile, compared to the alternative, if it had much higher effectiveness. Nevertheless, some branded products may offer only marginal advantages over much cheaper generics.

It can be seen, therefore, that the choice of drug is not a simple matter. Certainly, greater efficiency would not be achieved by the use of the cheapest available product in each case. Thus, there is a clear role for economic evaluation in investigating the relative cost-effectiveness of prescribing options. Some studies have already been undertaken (Drummond, Teeling Smith and Wells 1988) and others are in progress. It is unrealistic to expect GPs to fund such studies, although some have been undertaken by central government (Anderson 1989). It is much more likely that the pharmaceutical industry will support such analysis as it perceives its interests as being threatened (Drummond 1989/90).

Discussion: What monitoring arrangements are required to ensure efficiency?

One of the main objectives of the White Paper proposals is to increase the efficiency of the NHS. Many of the right kinds of incentives will be put in place, but will decision-makers respond by carefully considering their options within an economic evaluation framework, or will they respond in a more *ad hoc* manner? That is, it may be easier to agree a price for a contract for clinical services than to assess cost or cost-effectiveness. This final section outlines the monitoring arrangements that will be required to ensure that important efficiency issues are being considered carefully by DHAs and FPCs. They could quite easily form part of the agenda for the annual review of these institutions in their new roles.

First, analysis should be carried out of how Health Authorities decide which contracts to place. Will this be based on historical precedent, or will a real effort be made to consider which investments in health care will give the best value for money? What, if any, analysis will support such decision-making processes.

Second, contract specifications (and successful contracts) should be scrutinised in order to assess how carefully the purchaser has specified the requirements and whether there is any evidence that, through the contracting process, cost-effective medical technologies are being encouraged. For example, is day-case surgery specified where this would be appropriate, or is the choice of treatment technology left to the provider?

Third, the processes by which HAs review contracts should be assessed. In particular, what attitudes do HAs take to contract deviations in respect of the cost, volume and quality of care?

Fourth, the approaches used by FPCs to promote cost-effective prescribing should be monitored. For example, in stimulating the development of community formularies, or in setting indicative budgets, do they take a broad view of cost (beyond the price of the medicines themselves) and do they consider the relative effectiveness of medicines?

Fifth, the efforts made by FPCs to promote cost-effective behaviour by those GPs opting to manage their own budgets should be monitored. For example, do they support GPs wishing to develop cost-effective alternatives to hospital admission and do they help GPs find the best value for money alternatives in placing contracts with hospitals for non-emergency admissions.

Clearly, the proposals in the White Paper represent the most fundamental change in the NHS since its inception. Others have highlighted the need for monitoring the changes brought about by the proposals (Judge 1989). Since one of the major objectives of the White Paper is to increase the efficiency of the NHS, it is important that health care objectives are evaluated from an economic viewpoint and that monitoring arrangements are put in place to ensure that HAs and FPCs rise to the challenge. This paper has outlined the ways of assessing efficiency, the ways in which the White Paper proposals present new opportunities and the monitoring arrangements to ensure that HAs and FPCs seize them.

References

Akehurst RL 1989 'What clinicians can contribute to option appraisal?' in Akehurst RL and Drummond MF (eds) *Clinicians as the Managers of Health Care Resources* National Health Service Training Authority, Bristol

Akehurst RL and Drummond MF 1989 *Clinicians as the Managers of Health Care Resources* National Health Service Training Authority, Bristol

Anderson RL 1989 *Economics of cholesterol measurement*. Presentation given at the Kings Fund Consensus Conference on the Measurement of Cholesterol, London, 26–28 June

Buxton MJ *et al.* 1985 *Costs and Benefits of the Heart Transplant Programme at Harefield and Papworth Hospital* HMSO, London

Central Birmingham Health Authority 1989 *Annual Report of the Department of Public Health*. CBHA Birmingham

Crump B, Drummond MF and Marchment M 1990 'The DGM's dilemma' *Health Service Journal* 12 April, 552–3

Davies LM, Drummond ME, Woodward EG and Buckley RJ 1986 'A cost-effectiveness comparison of the intraocular lens and contact lens in aphakia' *Transactions of the Ophthalmological Society of the United Kingdom* **105**, 3, 304–13

Department of Health 1989a *Working for patients* DoH, London

Department of Health 1989b *Primary Health Care Services* DoH, London

Department of Health 1989c *Funding General Practice* Dec DoH, London

Department of Health and Social Security 1981 *Health Services Management. Health Building Projects* HN (81) 30, DHSS, London

Department of Health and Social Security 1983 *Performance Indicators for the NHS* DHSS, London

Department of Health and Social Security (1988) *Option Appraisal of Medical and Scientific Equipment* HMSO, London

Department of Health 1990 *Operating Contracts* DoH, London

Drummond MF 1980 *Principles of Economic Appraisal in Health Care* Oxford Medical Publications, Oxford

Drummond MF 1988 'Economics aspects of cataract' *Ophthalmology* **95**, 8, 1147–53

Drummond MF 1989 'The economics of drug formularies' *Pharmaceutical Journal* 15 April, 451–2

Drummond MF 1989/90 'The role of economic evaluation in the pricing of modern pharmaceutical products' *Pharmaceutical Times* Dec, Jan, Feb, Mar

Drummond MF 1990 'Will competition drive out quality?' in *Quality and Contracts* Hereford, National Association for Quality Assurance in Health Care

Drummond MF and Hutton 1987

Drummond MF, Stoddart DL and Torrance GW 1987 *Methods for the Economic Evaluation of Health Care Programmes* Oxford University Press, Oxford

Drummond MF and Maynard AK 1988 'Efficiency in the NHS: lessons from abroad' *Health Policy* **9**, 83–96

Drummond MF, Teeling Smith G and Wells N 1988 *Economic Evaluation in the Development of Medicines* Office of Health Economics, London

Drummond MF and Yates JM 1988 'Clearing the cataract backlog in a not-so-developing country' *Report for the National Eye Institute* Methesda, MD

Drummond MF, Marchment M and Crump B 1989 'Taking the bit between your teeth' *Health Service Journal* 14 Sep, 1126–8

Drummond MF and McGuire A 1990 'The economics of lipid-lowering drugs' in Lewis B *et al.* (eds) *The Social and Economic Contexts of Coronary Heart Disease Prevention* Current Medical Literature, London

Evans RG 1985 *Strained Mercy: the Economics of the Canadian Health Care System* Butterworths, New York

Graham DY, Agrawal NW and Roth SH 1988 'Prevention of NSAID-induced gastric ulcer with misoprostol: multicentre, double-blind placebo-controlled trial' *Lancet* **11**, 1277–80

Inter-authority Comparisons and Consultancy (IACC) 1989 *Examining some of England's Longest Waiting Lists: Half Year Report* Health Services Management Centre, Birmingham, IACC

Judge K 1989 'Monitoring and evaluating working for patients' *British Medical Journal* **299**, 1385–7

Labelle RJ 1987 'Planning for the provision and utilization of new health care technologies' in Feeny D, Guyatt G and Tugwell P (eds) *Health Care Technology: Effectiveness, Efficiency and Public Policy* Institute for Research on Public Policy, Halifax (NS)

Ludbrook A and Mooney GH 1983 *Economic Appraisal in the NHS* Northern Health Economics, Aberdeen

Maxwell R 1985 *Health and Wealth* Lexington Books, DC Heath & Co, Lexington

Russell IT, Devlin HB, Fell M *et al.* 1977 'Day-care surgery for hernias and haemorrhoids: a clinical, social and economic evaluation' *Lancet* 844–7

Thomas HF, Darvell RHJ and Hicks C 1989 '"Operation cataract": a means of reducing waiting lists for cataract operations' *British Medical Journal* **299**, 961–3

University of York 1990 *Health Economics at York* York

Waller J *et al.* 1978 *Early Discharge from Hospital for Patients with Hernia or Varicose Veins* HMSO, London

Ware J *et al.* 1986 Comparison of Health Outcomes of a Health Maintenance Organisation with those of Free-for-service' *Lancet* **1**, 1017–22

Warner KE and Luce BR 1982 *Cost-benefit and Cost-effectiveness analysis in Health Care* Health Administration Press, Ann Arbor (MI)

Williams AH 1985 'Economics of coronary artery bypass grafting' *British Medical Journal* **291**, 326–9

Yates JM and Davidge M 1984 'Can you measure performance?' *British Medical Journal* **288**, 77–83

5 Resource management: a fundamental change in managing health services

Peter Spurgeon

The NHS reforms have provoked, and continue to provoke, widespread and heated debate. In both the political arena and in the public domain reactions have been sharply divided. In particular the establishment of self-governing Trusts, service contracts and GP fundholding has proved contentious and controversial. Many of these issues are discussed within this text. This wider ranging debate has achieved a high profile and rather overshadowed the resource management initiative. Ironically purchaser/provider relationships and more detailed contract specifications rely upon the development of the sort of information and organisational structures implicit in resource management systems. The latter initiative in the longer term may well prove to be the most fundamental change of all in the way that health services are managed.

The Resource Management Initiative (RMI) is of course rather less new since it was formally announced in 1986. The key stated aim was to enable 'the NHS to give better service to its patients by helping clinicians and other managers to make better informed judgements about how the resources they control can be used to the maximum effect'. The assumption of the reforms that resource management systems are up and running, and fully operational is still some way off in many units.

Considerable confusion still exists about just what is meant by RMI, what does it entail and what are the benefits to the patient? Discussions about RMI tend to produce a range of concepts and confusions. Clinicians in particular have been guarded in their enthusiasm about becoming embroiled in management and expressing concerns as to whether their involvement represents the best use of their time. Perhaps more cynically some clinicians are uneasy about activity and cost information being used to further control their clinical freedom. General doubts have been expressed about the cost of introducing resource management and whether this money might not have been deployed more effectively on direct patient care. In response to this concern the Management Executive in 1992 have issued a manual aimed at estimating the costs of establishing resource management systems.

In some ways of course the differing views about RMI are quite healthy because RMI is not a single entity, nor is there a single way of implementing RMI. As Packwood, Keen and Buxton (1992) describe units have adopted quite different patterns of organisation and implementation reinforcing the view that RMI is an approach to managing health services rather than the application of a specific system.

The aim of this chapter is to explore the nature of RMI, to understand some of the key elements (information systems, organisational and cultural change) and to examine the impact of RMI on managerial processes.

The basics of RMI

As an earlier chapter discussing financial aspects of health care has made clear RMI is not new. It evolved as an idea from a previous initiative in 1983 known as management budgeting. Lack of appropriate data systems, lack of involvement of clinicians and a basically top-down, finance led approach did not result in a great deal of success for this initiative. RMI has been able to benefit from this experience, in part fortuitously because of the progress in information technology. More critical though was the clear indication that the key resource allocators, ie doctors and nurses, must be an integral part of developing any such approach. Not only must the users of such a system find the data relevant and credible, they must also be motivated to use it to improve the overall performance of their activities. Here is the key to successful RMI and a hint as to the major cultural change that is implied. Both these aspects will be discussed later in some depth.

A further advantage of RMI over previous approaches was that it was consistent with the growing influence of general management. Some general managers had been rather unfairly linked with cost containment and cut-backs. To some degree managers do have a responsibility to control costs or rather to optimise the use of available resources. Managers and clinicians had rather come to view each other as protagonists in the constant battle for resources. 'Patients must come first' has always been the rallying cry of the clinicians, almost as if for managers the opposite held true. However, RMI offered a way of integrating the two perspectives so that the measurement of service quality and the effective control of costed inputs could finally be brought together. The opportunity presented by RMI is nicely summed up in a paper by Black, Dearden, Mathew and Nichol (1989) in which they say 'Resource management enables clinicians and managers to see directly what the cost of various patterns of care are, to consider alternatives and make decisions in a more informed way – at the level of patient, the service or service mix. Visible connections between inputs, care, processes, outputs and the management of the whole can be of immense benefit to professionals and managers striving to make improvements against the odds'.

RMI may be summed up rather simplistically but powerfully as being about the linking of clinical activity data, for both volume and quality (at individual patient and case mix level) to resource utilisation such that costs can be identified on a projective basis. This statement is not quite the same as the official DHSS objectives for RMI but it represents a reasonable paraphrasing. The key objectives of the DHSS are essentially:

1. the medical and nursing groups must have a genuine sense of ownership in the management process;

2. improved quality of patient care;

3. patient case mix and costing systems must be evolved to allow for comparisons of resource utilisation; and

4. the accuracy of basic patient activity data must be improved so that it commands the confidence of the user.

These statements, if fully operationalised, represent a major cultural change in the way health services are managed. For the first time the system will be capable of identifying just what it is doing (activities) and what each element of the process costs. This of course is almost the natural management approach of the private sector, exemplified by the manufacturing industry where output of products and costs of manufacture are absolutely crucial information. Many have and will continue to argue that the private sector model cannot be transferred to health care. Indeed Spurgeon and Barwell (1990) have raised a number of queries as to the appropriateness of utilising management processes relevant to one situation in a totally different context. Nevertheless it seems in the light of pressures for greater public accountability that the health service cannot mount a credible argument as to why it should not be clear about just what activities it is performing and what they cost. It is important though that the fears of clinicians who see such information as a threat and prelude to increasing cost containment are addressed. The same data if used properly can offer a more exciting challenge of ensuring that the most cost-effective decisions are taken and actually enhance patient care rather than reduce it. The access to data about treatment outcome and quality of care should be a major incentive for clinicians. Those responsible for implementing RMI need to ensure that it is these latter opportunities that are projected and not an attack on clinical judgement.

The manner of implementing RMI on a national level is through a series of phased programmes. An initial set of six acute sites were identified as pilots for RMI beginning in 1987, although one was not formally adopted as a pilot site until 1988. Following this group a further twenty units were identified for the next group and these twenty came from within a batch of fifty who will form the subsequent groups, and so on through the service. Clearly one of the potential advantages of this approach is that successive RMI implementations can learn the lessons of earlier sites and hopefully avoid problems and thus speed up the total process. As part of this learning exercise a team from Brunel University was asked to monitor and evaluate the first six field sites. An interim report (Buxton, Packwood and Keen) was published in 1989, with a final report by Packwood, Keen and Buxton in 1991. Rather than consider comments on each individual site some more general points about RMI overall may be made.

Implementing RMI

One particularly helpful observation made by the reports was the identification of three key features which although not exactly pre-scriptions for success are certainly aspects that need to be incorporated. The first of these concerns management arrangements and is concerned with how far organisational structures facilitate the RMI process in terms of issues such as ownership, accountability, incentives and support to users. The second area is located around the development of information systems involving considerations such as meaningfulness, accuracy and accessibility of data. The third and final category is almost a superordinate to the other two in that it asks how all the changes implied in the first two aspects are being handled.

The value of the structure lies in indicating that parallel progress on all fronts is an important ingredient of successful implementation. Approaches that have tended to over emphasise the cost aspects of RMI and to make it appear as a finance driven system tend to alienate the service provider groups and often meet with resistance at clinician level. Similarly an over-emphasis upon bringing doctors into the management process can lead to frustration if good reliable sources of information delivery are not being developed at the same time. However it is equally clear that no single organisational structure has evolved as the correct one for supporting RMI. This was always intended to be the case as each unit adopted components of RMI systems and shaped the organisation to their own special needs. Grasping this notion of parallel development on all fronts can alleviate many of the misconceptions about RMI. In this way RMI does not become about computer systems, or medical audit or about attaching costs to everything. RMI must be an integrated process or it is likely to fail.

Does this mean therefore that RMI has to be a massive concentrated effort to bring everything on-stream at the same time? This approach, often labelled the 'big bang' approach, is not essential and indeed can be counterproductive. Individuals can be overawed by the thought of the very large system, it can appear to be totally dominated by technology and moreover it is expensive. It is of course quite possible to develop an integrated system based on a single hardware base. The key to success with such an approach is planning and communication such that everyone involved understands what is happening and their own role within the total picture.

Many sites have advanced on an incremental basis by developing one area on a small scale system. This too is entirely reasonable but it does require that attention be paid to compatibilities of systems so that future system integration remains possible.

One begins to see why some staff are confused by RMI. For example seeing a desk top PC arrive on the unit general manager's desk – is this RMI? Or others may be asked to participate in lengthy discussions about what information needs they have – if this is RMI where is the computer? It all serves to emphasise the point that RMI is an approach, or process of management and all these elements have a part to play but in a co-ordinated, integrated fashion.

Let us examine what lessons have been learned about RMI from existing sites and also what are the emerging issues that the service will need to tackle to make the most of the opportunities offered by RMI.

Managing the organisational and cultural transition

In the past the NHS has perhaps been guilty of seeing structures and organisational change as the outcome measures of new initiatives. The fallacy of course in this thinking is that any organisational structure is the means not the end. Therefore, whatever arrangements evolve they should have as an underlying principle of their design the goal that they will assist the organisation or unit to achieve its objective. The initial and overriding goal in terms of RMI is to ensure that the service providers (doctors, nurses, other professional groups) are fully integrated into the management process. To a large extent the discussion has centred around bringing doctors into management and perhaps as the primary and key resource allocator this is appropriate. It is important however that the other groups do not feel either overlooked or subservient to the medical power base.

Despite the emphasis laid by the Griffiths Report (1983) on the need to involve doctors in management the degree of success in this respect was until quite recently very limited. For many general managers the key to their own success was either how to involve doctors and obtain co-operation or how to overcome intransigence from doctors when trying to bring about change. The Templeton series on district general managers confirmed the importance of this issue but also the lack of progress.

The traditional system for involvement of clinicians tends to have been based upon some element of divisional structures with different specialities coming together as a representative body as the Medical Executive Committee. Although the MECs were often influential bodies and had a valuable information role they were not typically felt to be good decision-making bodies enabling doctors to make prompt and positive contributions to management. Some of the initial RMI pilot sites utilised arrangements based around this traditional structure, with medical staff committees playing a representative role. As the purchaser/provider separation has proceeded and specific contracts have been placed so it has become necessary to evolve to smaller speciality based structures.

In most RMI contexts this new structure has become almost universally a version of the clinical directorate model. This concept was originally pioneered at the Johns Hopkins Hospital, Baltimore in 1973 and consisted of a medical director supported by a nurse and an administrator. In the UK the concept of the administrator has been replaced by the term 'business manager' and 'the medical director'.

There is a natural logic to such a structure in that management can reasonably be said to be about making the best use of the resources available and to this extent is a normal part of the clinical process. Individual clinicians are constantly taking management decisions. Indeed Horsley, Vaughan, Hessetter and Allen (1989) argue that consultants are always involved in management at different levels – patient, staff, representing colleagues. Many clinicians are therefore suitable to make the transition into management implied by the directorate structure. Moreover management issues do arise naturally when clinicians work together in teams, perhaps with nurses and other professional staff. Judgements about staffing requirements, levels of workload, achievable standards and so on require managerial as well as clinical skills. The idea of the clinical directorate is that the groupings of service providers can be given responsibility for organising their work including its planning and budgeting control. The aims of the clinical directorate structure may be described as follows:

1. Accountability – many of the changes in the NHS over recent years have had an implicit if not explicit goal of strengthening the notion of line management. Unit and individual accountability, IPR, Regional review and performance indicators are all in this mould. However, the traditional position of the doctor does not fit well the concept of line management in that the greatest power, expertise and control rests with the 'worker' not management. The clinical directorate model seeks to rectify this by equating authority with responsibility, power with accountability.

2. Decentralisation – by delegating responsibility and authority for operational decision-making and resultant resource consumption implications to the appropriate level of service delivery the clinical directorate structure seeks to improve the quality of that decision-making. The service-specific-disciplinary management team is in the best position to make well-informed decisions. In addition it provides the logical level at which to undertake quality assessment, audit and utilisation review activities.

3. Clinical efficiency – monitoring the cost-effectiveness of resource consumption is clearly central to the theory underlying the development of the structure. By placing responsibility for costs in the hands of clinicians expenditure control can be made more sensitive to the clinical priorities. As many clinicians will point out, utilisation review at its best should be as much about good clinical practice (ie clinical efficiency) as about cost containment.

4. Focus – clinical directorates offer a management structure that is based on the delivery of a given service to a group of clients. This is in contrast to the traditional structure based upon professional hierarchies. This in turn provides a basis for analysis of case-mix and volume and their subsequent management.

The Brunel report suggests that where clinical directorates are not in place then a transitional slightly diluted form of clinical groupings exists. The key difference is that in the latter form there is limited meaningful budgetary devolution into the groupings with unit management teams largely retaining varying degrees of central financial control.

Many clinicians have seized the opportunities implicit within the clinical directorate grouping structure believing that in a cash limited system the most positive response to any threat to clinical freedom is to become involved in the discussions stemming from the financial restriction (Stuart, Spurgeon and Cook in the press). A rather sophisticated version of this view is that RMI represents a legitimisation of the tension and debate between managers and clinicians as to who shall have the dominant perspective. All professionals will have as an objective the desire to provide a service to their client at the highest possible standard using whatever resources may be required. The corporate objectives of managers may often appear in conflict with this and hence the tension between the two groups. RMI will be about the quality, quantity and cost of services to be delivered and hence provides the perfect vehicle for the debate between clinician and manager to be conducted and resolved. The critical step is for clinicians to be willing to enter the arena and to participate.

Just how is this participation to be ensured? One approach that seems appealing at a commonsense level is to facilitate the evolution of natural groups of clinicians who work together because their specialties and interests are common. These individuals can then form the basis of a directorate with a positive desire and will to coordinate since it will clearly be seen as a way of enhancing their effectiveness. Moreover, as in the pilot sites such groups might initially be encouraged to develop the concept of quality profiles for individual patients. In effect these become projected standards of care and treatments that attach to patients of a particular group. Not only does this allow the clinical group to monitor and modify their own treatment programmes but subsequently through the introduction of costing systems enable clinicians and managers to come together to plan case mix and future service patterns.

Overall the clear conclusion is that RMI prompts, perhaps requires, some form of sub-unit structure to emerge. In terms of the objectives of RMI this is entirely consistent, since sub-unit structures become the focus of devolution, decentralisation and the appropriate focus for decisions and debates about resource utilisation. Moreover, this organisational structure is a natural outcome of more general reforms where contracts are focussed upon specialties or collectives of specialties. It is at sub unit level that issues of quality, medical audit and cost control will really be tackled. Once again the implicit linkage of the RMI as a fundamental basis of wider reforms is made explicit.

Despite the rapid growth of clinical directorates and clinically based management structures there is remarkably little research about how the transition from clinician to manager is being supported, or the degree of success achieved. The individualistic perspective of doctors as opposed to the more collective approach of managers has already been mentioned. Fitzgerald and Sturt (1992), after further valuable insights into difficulties of handling the transition, point to a lack of clarity about the roles of clinical directors and the assumptions doctors tend to hold about the learning process. For many doctors management is a technical procedure to be read about and acquired in much the same way as many of the factually based aspects of medical education. The experiential basis of much management learning can feel alien.

Willcocks (1992) adds further evidence to these concerns reporting that many doctors feel confused and disillusioned about their management role. He suggests that this is in part about lack of role clarity, but also about a lack of support in acquiring a broad understanding of the culture of NHS management. It is likely that these difficulties will intensify as the clinical management role becomes not just operational but strategic as well involving debates with purchasers about potentially radical changes in service patterns and delivery style. Purchasers in the 1993–4 round of contracts will be seeking savings targets which may ultimately be obtainable only by revised service patterns within directorates. It remains to be seen how far clinical directors will be content to be part of significant changes that may affect the clinical practice of their medical colleagues.

Issues surrounding clinical directorates

The basic model is one of a clinical director (usually a clinician) responsible managerially for the operational work of all the staff within the directorate. Assistance is typically provided by a nurse manager and by a business manager; these 'assistants' have concerns with the collection and interpretation of information, the planning and monitoring of directorate activity.

An immediate potential problem arises regarding a possible ethical infringement upon the doctor–patient relationship. This could be a dilemma for both the clinical director and other consultants within the directorate. For the latter group there may be concerns as to how they can accept being responsible and accountable to another doctor in their dealings with patients. Whilst for the director there exists possible conflict between maximising provision for patient care at an individual level and the need to monitor and control expenditure at a directorate level. Such concerns can create new and significant demands upon the staff management skills of new clinical directors. Indeed, it is for many a major adjustment since the prevailing medical culture suggests that once doctors acquire consultant status they are self-contained, autonomous individuals accountable to no one other than their patients. This is stated in a rather extreme manner to make the point. Nevertheless the notion of collective decision-making about patient care, about priorities and treatment options is quite alien.

There is of course much work to be done in the service as a whole to support and develop the skills of new clinical directors. Some early clinical directors might be considered 'natural managers' but a more planned provision of training in aspects such as service planning and review, objective setting, information handling, financial and staff management is required to ensure a continuity of appropriate clinical directors.

There are equally significant changes implied in the role of general managers. Chief Executives in particular must be willing to see real devolution of power to the directorates. Any sense that directorates are a mechanism to control and constrain doctors is likely to provoke problems. For some UGMs this change will be threatening, especially as, with the advent of contracts for services, some Districts toy with the idea of placing contracts directly with the clinical director, effectively by-passing the Unit Manager. This, though, is unlikely to be the norm and there is a challenge to Chief Executives to re-define their role and relationship to a series of clinical directors. An enhanced coordinating role is available to those capable of meeting this challenge, especially as the number of Districts and Units reduces and Chief Executives come to represent larger conglomerations of provider groupings.

Perhaps even more vociferous concerns have been expressed by nurses and paramedic groups who fear the medical domination of the current structuring of clinical directorates. Despite, in many instances, retained professional lines of accountability, the decision-making about resources to deliver nursing care or to engage paramedic services lies with the director. Under financial pressure the concern is that a clinical director may seek to contain his/her budget by cuts in such support services. A recent paper by Norman, Quinn and Malin (1988) expresses concern as to the degree of involvement of nurses in the resource management process. A key aspect for nurses in particular, but for RMI overall, is that progress be made on the concept of collaborative care plans whereby the whole team agree a pattern of treatment, and therefore resources, that will be needed by a particular patient. The advent of more examples of non-medical clinical directors may well reduce this concern, as will the development of specific service contracts where each group will have committed to buying or providing an agreed package of care and support.

Despite these issues the clinical model appears to be gaining ground as a basis for structures to support RMI. This is not surprising since experience at the pilot sites has thrown-up some important benefits and opportunities. Where directorate systems work well there seems to be an increase in staff morale and greater cooperation between professional groups as they cohere around an integrated programme of patient care. Furthermore the directorate provides the foundation for a cooperative problem solving approach involving clinicians and managers.

There appear to be some important challenges for sustaining and developing the concept further:

1. Maintaining corporate identity. Ironically as directorates become successful so there is a greater sense of identification and loyalty to the particular directorate rather than to the hospital unit. Such feelings can of course be very positive but must not develop to the extent that they produce an unhealthy rivalry and competitiveness. This issue is increasingly important as unit configurations change and the purchaser/provider distribution becomes more developed between DHA and provider units.

2. Adjusting to a more rational service planning process. As the process of contract specification develops and the role of public health expands so there exists the potential to alter current patterns of service to ones that may more appropriately reflect population need and assess outcome. This may prove a major challenge to clinicians expecting to carry on much as before.

3. Emphasising quality of care. RMI has as an objective the involvement of clinicians in management. This may or may not attract sufficient doctors to want to be involved. But what should stimulate the medical professions is the tremendous opportunity offered by RMI for medical audit and progress in assessing the quality of the service. Once again this is an issue that will be of increasing interest to purchasers.

4. Ensuring that the transition from clinician to manager is better supported and that the succession of consultants into future clinical directors is properly planned.

Developing information systems

The information area is another instance where RMI has become entangled and confused with a number of information initiatives in the NHS over the past few years. Again it is not totally inappropriate that this sort of overlap should exist since RMI must build upon the data that exists within the service; it cannot be separate and unrelated to that which currently exists.

Much has been said about the 'information revolution' in the NHS. More has been said than has actually happened. There are all sorts of contributory reasons for this situation although there is a steady pressure to change the future. Initially it is probably fair to say that the NHS has always been a prolific collector of data, usually fairly basic data and almost always for bureaucratic purposes to satisfy regional or national demands for returns. However, much less well developed has been the nature of using information for decision-making. Managers have not, on the whole, been predisposed to numerically oriented analysis, clinicians have not pushed for cost or outcome data preferring to focus upon patient care processes and cash inputs have been on the basis of fairly crude recurring allocations.

Cash limits have prompted increasing efforts to determine the sources of particular expenditure and there have been initiatives in the financial area to decide whether to improve collection of descriptive information or to concentrate on cost-effectiveness programmes. Much of this has been rather narrow, confined to financial staff, and has therefore had limited impact upon managers and clinicians.

This rather piecemeal approach has been paralleled in terms of how the NHS has acquired hardware and software systems. Districts and Units have taken initiatives but often they have not been coordinated within a District and certainly not as a national service. Overall there has been no clear information strategy. Recently a number of initiatives have been launched to counteract this situation. In particular the NHS Management Board has developed an Information Management and Training Strategy (1989) which attempts to identify training and support requirements for staff within the NHS.

Regions too have attempted to develop their own information strategies. However, two overriding problems remain:

1. Too often technology becomes the dominant feature of information system development, frequently to the detriment of the resultant system.

2. Data proliferates in the NHS, with more and more being collected but without the same effort being put into asking why it is being collected and what it is to be used for.

Thus we have a situation where data is not transformed into information. What staff need is information that addresses a specific need or objective of their job, and what typically they receive is a mass of data not properly tailored to their needs and so difficult to penetrate that it falls into disuse.

The primary need when dealing with the information issue is to establish clearly what various staff need to do their jobs and then to see how to provide this more limited selection of information in a form that is easily available and accessible.

A number of approaches exist for helping to determine information requirements, for example Task Analysis (Spurgeon and Barwell 1989) which is a technique that moves from a statement of work objectives to an identification of the information needs that underpin these tasks. RMI needs to ensure, in the way that it tackles the information aspect, that it can incorporate properly the 'user led' aspect of information specification. This approach of course has the added and considerable value of involving the users of the systems (doctors, nurses, managers) in specifying what they want to get from it. Not only is this likely to increase the likelihood of relevance of the information it also enhances user commitment. Furthermore there exists the prospect that through this approach RMI could acquire a proper emphasis on the quality and outcome of patient care.

There is a danger that this opportunity may be missed. Of the initial pilot sites relatively little progress was made in terms of collecting outcome information. In part this was a result of the relatively early stages of RMI but it is an aspect that must be addressed and addressed with a sense of priority. In addition, as Coombs and Cooper (1990) stress in their report, unless sufficient involvement of clinicians is ensured in developing the system then, often by default, the result is a finance-led system. Their view is that this will lead to clinical resistance and ultimately a failure to implement.

Most of the existing pilot sites opted for a fairly large scale computer based system with a central system that stores, for case mix purposes, the data from a number of locally based feeder units. A 'core' of data was defined by existing systems, eg pathology, theatres, although of course with some site variation. Once again the potential for data as opposed to information is in operation. One is beginning with what exists not what is needed. Of course the latter will relate and feed off the wider data base but good systems development practice says that this should be identified at the outset. In fact the emphasis of the pilot sites appears to have been on activity data as supplied through operational units. Surprisingly little has been done on identifying the needs of managers. It is important that the managerial information does not become seen as equivalent to cost data, otherwise there is the inevitable perception that managers simply want information to control costs. Managers have a much wider opportunity than this since good information should enable them, virtually for the first time, to have a valid input in the pattern of the service within a unit for which they are responsible. Considerable support is required to help managers see how they can analyse and utilise RMI information for more effective decision making.

One of the key features of RMI must be the capacity for clinicians, nurses or the clinical directorate to identify prospective care plans. These will in effect be a statement of the treatment and care a patient should receive with associated standards attached. An essential ingredient of this is the ability to categorise each patient by disease type or treatment group. The typical approach to this problem is to utilise some version of the DRG (Diagnostic Related Group). Jenkins, McKee and Sanderson (1990) describe DRGs as one form of classificatory scheme for hospital inpatients. Each patient belongs to one group only and this is determined by his/her principal diagnosis and/or surgical operation, in conjunction with factors such as age and sex. The concept of DRGs was developed in the USA and some British clinicians have been critical of their appropriateness, at least believing that more work is needed to make them usable in the NHS.

The DRG structure is one of many systems available. Views differ as to suitability of various systems and it may well be that different systems and models emerge. It is a matter of conjecture as to how far the prospect of different classificatory structures will ultimately prevent the sort of comparisons such systems are meant to facilitate. There is a danger that the size of the NHS will again produce a range of systems and subsequently years of argument as to whether the data deriving from one system can truly be compared with another system because the items included are not common or are not grouped in the same way. It is a situation which cries out for centralised resolution of the type the large commercial organisation can impose. It is unlikely to be forthcoming in the NHS.

Nevertheless some sort of classificatory scheme to group patient types seems to be essential. In essence such schemes should facilitate the following positive aspects:

1. examination of treatment patterns and associated costs;

2. examination of variations in case mix between hospitals, specialties and/or consultants.

But perhaps the key aspect that will appeal to doctors in considering DRGs is their contribution to medical audit. As long as proper outcome data are collected there is clearly scope for care to be at the forefront of discussion of RMI. This seems the appropriate priority to attract resource users to participate in developing such a system. Whilst the potential here looks considerable there is just a slight concern that initial reaction has been that medical audit requires a rather more in depth review of each case than is provided by routine data collection approaches. Furthermore Maynard (1991) has pointed to concerns about DRGs as cost pricing systems without having equally clear statements about quality of care. The latter may prove difficult to achieve until good data is available both on outcome and on a more subtle classification of initial severity of the case.

The very word 'routine' as mentioned earlier highlights some of the initial teething problems of RMI systems. As with all information systems the effectiveness is largely dependent upon the quality of data entering the system. The susceptibility of coders handling large quantities of technical data is self-evident. In the USA where RMI type systems have gone much further the quality of coders is very high. It is not surprising then that training initiatives have been launched to support and develop medical records staff in the UK.

Alongside this training need is the concern about the shortage of high quality information technology staff to develop and monitor the progress of RMI systems. The ultimate success of RMI on a national basis may depend upon the recruitment of such staff and subsequently their ability to provide information in an accurate way and in the form specified by the ultimate system user.

Managing change

The previous two aspects are clearly the main thrusts of RMI but combining them together successfully and reducing negative fall-out within the organisation is in effect the third aspect, that of managing the cultural change that new systems will inevitably produce. There are many texts on organisational change and this is not the appropriate place to develop these theoretical models (see Spurgeon and Barwell 1990). Nevertheless, implementing RMI is going to change the culture of the NHS and recognising this means that there is almost certain to be resistance.

There may in some instances be local 'champions' who are willing to lead and to encourage others to participate. Obviously where these exist it is important to use the opportunity and to consider how they can best be integrated with the more reluctant mass. Failing this there are still things that managers can do. Broadly, these roles fall into two main areas, communication and training.

Communication

The roles of some key staff are likely to be affected by RMI and this may be perceived as a threat. It is essential that everyone is kept informed about what is involved and just how the new system will impact upon them. In this way individual operations can be shaped to be realistic rather than at odds with the likely outcome. Similarly the relationship between staff, notably doctors and managers, may change with new senses of power and control developing. Only by involving every group in the evolution of these structures can problems be avoided.

Training

Information technology is in itself threatening to many. Acquisition of basic skills throughout a department needs to be planned and phased such that new systems are online with individual staff feeling comfortable and confident of their abilities to cope. Any hint of difficulties is likely to spread and make others resist the onset of the 'new fangled' equipment.

Allied to this is the appropriate acquisition of resources both human and technical, to support the developments. Once again the phasing of this support is vital to the smooth introduction of information systems.

Finally, Mathew (1989) drawing upon Canadian experience suggests that the management of cultural change is the key to utilising resource management as an agent of improved health care for patients. He lists some vital organisational factors in creating this positive perception:

1. commitment to patient care and resource management must be emphasised as mutually supportive goals;

2. resource management must be demonstrated to be linked to a client orientation, hence the criticality of involving users in specifying care and quality parameters;

3. the information resulting from resource management must be seen as an open system available to be discussed in a safe atmosphere but one which seeks for improvements.

In conclusion, this chapter has presented a case for RMI being a fundamental change in the way health care is managed. It represents a tremendous opportunity and challenge but these will only be obtained if the development of organisational change and information systems is properly integrated and managed. There is mounting pressure within the NHS via the information demands of the reforms to implement RM systems. Contract monitoring, quality specifications and the requirement to provide purchasers (both DHA and GP fundholders) with prices (based on accurate costings) all require provider organisations to supply good information. Beyond the information the organisations must also be structurally equipped to deliver their contracts. It is in this way that RMI becomes totally integrated and fundamental to the wider reforms of the NHS.

References

Black A, Dearden R, Mathew D and Nichol D 1989 *The Extension of Resource Management: An Audit for Action*. NHSTA Bristol

Buxton M, Packwood T and Keen J 1989 *Resource Management: Process and Progress*. Department of Health

Coombs R and Cooper D 1990 *Accounting for Patients: Information Technology and the Implementation of the NHS White Paper*. Policy Research Paper, UMIST Manchester

DHSS 1983 *NHS Management Inquiry (Griffiths Report). HMSO London*

Fitzgerald L and Sturt J 1992 'Clinicians into management: on the change agenda or not' *Health Services Management Research* **5**, 2, 137–146

Horsley SD, Vaughan DH, Hessetter C and Allen DEC 1989 'Management for consultants' *Journal of Management in Medicine* **4**, 4, 272–276

Jenkins L, McKee M and Sanderson H 1990 *DRGs. A Guide to Grouping and Interpretation.* CASPE research London

Mathew D 1989 'Providing excellent patient care with resource management' *Journal of management in medicine* **4**, 4, 267–271

Maynard A 1991 'Is there a future for a competitive health care market in Europe? An appraisal of the situation in England' in Kostoulis J (ed.) *The Future of Competitive Health Care in Europe.* Erasmus University Rotterdam

NHSME 1992 *Revenue Consequences of Resource Management*

NHSTA Bristol 1988 *Information Management and Technology Strategy*

Norman S, Quinn H and Malin H 1988 *The Resource Management Initiative and Ward Nursing Management Information Systems* Report by the Department of Health Nursing Division and Operational Research Services, London

Packwood T, Keen J and Buxton M 1991 *Hospitals in Transition: The Resource Management Experiment.* Open University Press

Packwood T, Keen J and Buxton M 1992 'Process and structure: resource management and the development of sub-unit organisational structure' *Health Services Management Research* **5**, 1, 66–76

Spurgeon P and Barwell F 1989 *The role of Analytic Techniques in Identification of Information Needs.* Health Services Management Centre Research Report 25

Spurgeon P and Barwell F 1990 *Implementing Change in the NHS: A Practical Guide for Managers.* Chapman and Hall, London

Stuart J, Spurgeon P and Cook AN (in the press) 'Making finance work for you' *British Medical Journal*

Willcocks SG 1992 'The role of the clinical director in the NHS: some observations' *Journal of Management in Medicine* **6**, 4, 41–46

6 Developing managers for the 1990s

David Thompson

Managers and development

The central theme of this chapter is that the challenge of developing managers for the 1990s is posed by the changing nature of NHS management itself. While management development can, and should, influence management, it will only be successful if it responds to the state of management. This vital factor was most clearly recognised by policy-makers in the 1980s:

> *If management is clear and confident about its purpose and tasks, the climate for management development is favourable. If management is confused or harassed, tired or demoralised, management development is an uphill task.* (Williams 1988)

In this context, management development can be seen to be any learning experience undergone by *those holding managerial roles in an organisation.* Such experience may be a highly visible educational programme, with recognised qualifications although no specified organisational outcome; it may be a training event focussed on particular skills and understanding; it may be an almost unrecognised flash of insight at the workplace, prompted consciously or unconsciously by others. It is well to share this perception that *learning* is at the heart of development because, even after nearly three decades of activities in the NHS, development is still associated by many managers with 'going on courses'. There is much more to it than that.

If development is the heart, the managerial organisation forms the skeleton. As the NHS enters the mid-1990s its organisation can be seen to be undergoing a 'third wave' of change. The first wave occurred after 1974, when a comprehensive change established an integrated structure within which the service could be efficiently administered. The intention was that managers should provide a positive and supportive climate for professionals to deliver health care. This traditional view has been summed up as follows:

> *The efficient control of expenditure is the cardinal management virtue. Those who pursue this approach tend to be relatively unconcerned with changes in the social and economic environment. They will implement policies but take few initiatives themselves. Their view of management rests on the assumption that a consensus exists on values and priorities within the Service. (NHS Training Authority 1986)*

The Griffiths Report, published in 1983, heralded the onset of the second wave. This was characterised by the assertion that management is concerned with:

> *levels of service, quality of product, meeting budgets, cost improvements, productivity, motivating and rewarding staff, research and development, and the long-term viability of the undertaking. (DHSS 1983)*

Griffiths found that the absence of 'general management support' meant that there was no driving force 'seeking and accepting direct and personal responsibility for developing plans, securing implementation and monitoring actual achievement'. This constituted an altogether more active management, which had to concern itself with professional matters.

These two waves were not, of course, neatly divided in time. The general management approach of the second wave was recognised and practised by some managers some time before the appearance of the Griffiths recommendations, especially after the structural 'tidying up' of 1982.

The flood tide of the third wave is now surging through the NHS as we approach the mid-1990s. It is now possible to evaluate its main features and to identify the implications for the development of managers.

A revolution about to happen?

Arguably, the most crucial event for the NHS in the decade so far has been the re-election of the Conservative Government in April 1992. This confirmed that the reforms proposed in the White Paper *Working for Patients* would continue to be implemented (DoH 1989a). NHS managers who had nailed their colours firmly to the fence before the general election were now able to plan changes within a framework whose main features were known. This news was good in so far as it reduced some of the political uncertainty surrounding the early part of 1992. Further good news came from the Government's anxiety to minimise disruption by ensuring a steady state and a smooth lift off in the early part of the implementation period. This gave some time to prepare an infrastructure. News which was less unqualifiably good was the lack of detail about important aspects of the new NHS. This constituted an opportunity for energetic managers to create their own response to the proposed internal market, while at the same time posing problems as policy makers and managers at all levels made their, sometimes contradictory, contributions to the debate.

At the time of writing, in mid-1993, the third wave of reform is now fairly launched: it will happen and is indeed happening. There is experiment with real change at all levels of the NHS. National politicians and policy makers are grappling with the problem of London's health care provision and world class medical centres. In fundholding practices throughout the land, general practitioners (GPs) are delivering measurably better services to their patients. In between, NHS managers are indulging in the game of managerial musical chairs which has been played during the re-structuring of the 1970s and 1980s. The difference this time round is that when the music stops, there will be fewer chairs for them to sit on.

The nagging doubt remains, however, that all the turmoil and changes will not add up to the promised revolution. It may be premature to harbour these doubts: the internal market has had scant chance to work. There are indeed signs that it is working, albeit in the crude way of all markets: senior managers and medical staff in many big city hospitals are coping with a dramatic shift in their traditional markets. But in retrospect, this may come to be seen as shifting the deckchairs on the secondary and tertiary decks of the NHS liner. Nearer the waterline, on the primary care deck, there are fewer signs of substantial change. It may yet come from GP fundholders if their enterprise continues to be backed, but it seems more likely that they will be financially and managerially reined in by the forces of 'accountability'.

What follows, then, should be read with the caution that the third wave may not carry us on its crest to the end of the millennium. It may be overtaken by a fourth wave whose proposals will be about a revolution in primary care, where the real health of the nation is delivered. Such speculation is not just abstract and academic: it has important implications for managers who must not become so absorbed in the implementation of the internal market that they close their minds to yet more and dramatic changes, even before the end of the decade.

Not withstanding this caution, the third wave of change has altered the face of the NHS management development in many ways. Six of the most significant are now discussed.

Provider development

The most striking feature of the White Paper reforms was the introduction of the purchaser–provider split which took effect in April 1991. This constitutes yet another attempt, following on those in 1974, 1982 and 1985, to delegate decision-making downwards. Previous efforts had always foundered on central insistence on 'accountability upwards', which effectively throttled any real local autonomy. This time round there are signs of greater success.

An increase in local autonomy is to come from the mechanism of the NHS Trust which could be established by any Unit or Units previously managing hospitals or community services under the direct control of a District Health Authority. After an uneasy couple of years it is now clear that all these NHS Units will become Trusts by April 1995. There has been a gestation period, unusually long even by NHS rates of change, because of uncertainties in national politics and of the need to prove financial and business viability.

The fog covering this new 'provider' landscape is now clearing, and some of the challenges for developing managers in the remainder of the 1990s are becoming evident. Much apparently remains the same as in the old days of 'management development', principally in the 1970s and 1980s. Hospitals did not change overnight in April 1991: they still consume great quantities of capital and revenue; they employ the majority of NHS staff and have a voracious appetite for supplies and information. They still require traditional skills of financial, human and information management: salaries and wages must be paid and accounted for; patients must be discharged and categorised. The skills to accomplish these important tasks – the life blood of the institutions – must be maintained and managers must still be developed to manage them.

These and additional competencies now however are in the valleys of the provider landscape. The high ground looks very different. It is not now a world of management in the old hierarchical sense, of a chain of command stretching from the ward sister and charge nurse to the Secretary of State. It is the world of the internal market. To be sure, this is not a market that the purists such as Kotler would recognise: it is not composed of two equal parties who are willing and able to trade something of value to each party (Kotler 1988). Le Grand describes it as a quasi-market, but a market nonetheless, in which consumers tend to be represented by agents and competition is not always between equals (Le Grand 1990).

Even the quasi-market has been slow and hesitant to arrive on the NHS scene. It may yet be prevented from operating by the political imperatives of public expenditure control and fierce 'provider' lobbying. But the impact so far constitutes undoubtedly the most important challenge to developing managers in this decade. It demands a whole new mind map for managers to navigate over the new landscape. They must be able to cope with a more fragmented world and one which recognises that the business of the NHS is now a business. The language of business would have been foreign to NHS managers even five years ago, but now it has percolated through even to many professionals who were accustomed to viewing their job as providing patient care to exact scientific standards with little attention to cost.

The language of business embraces the fact that NHS trusts have to operate in a fragmented NHS market, albeit with national and regional regulation. The focal point has become the business plan, the essential ingredient of the bid for trust status, and the blueprint for subsequent operations. The plan demands a consciousness of costs which transcends previous drives for value for money. This is still a new art, foreign to many professionals and traditional managers, as some of the more bizarre stabs at a pricing policy have revealed. At the same time, the trend towards an emphasis on quality has been absorbed into the business planning process. This must be an improvement on professional paternalism and the legacy of postwar 'austerity' welfarism but, again, there remains some way to go before the drive to improve quality becomes internalised within managers. All too often it arises from a response to external stimulus, such as the Patients' Charter. The quality assurance 'movement' in some ways reveals, and in other ways obscures, a greater awareness of the consumer – the patients, relatives and public of yesteryear. There have been some strides towards a better deal for the consumer: shorter waiting lists and waiting time, even better physical surroundings. But there remain severe conceptual and practical difficulties. The consumer can be seen to be both the payer – the purchasers – and the user – the patients – and the interests of these parties are often not identical. Indeed, they are often not known, because providers are accustomed to provide what provider professionals deem appropriate, and they have only the most rudimentary idea of what their users need, want and demand.

The market and its language show how a new reality in the outer world must become internalised into a new mind set. Old ways of thinking are clearly not sufficient: beds and budgets no longer matter; gaining the competitive edge is becoming all important. This is not comfortable for managers developed in the old NHS. But without the mental adjustment, they will find it difficult to absorb and use the related skills of market research and definition, negotiating and contracting.

The new language is, then, imperfectly understood. The task of developing managers to interpret and implement what it stands for is formidable. This constitutes a new agenda for the remainder of the decade and beyond. Comprehending the outer world of the market and the inner world of the new mind map are immediate development challenges. A further challenge for managers is converging and may come to dominate the final years of the decade. This will be the way in which people – NHS employees – are managed. The market has brought a cultural revolution which has profoundly affected chief executives and their directorial teams (for the most part). It is beginning to impact on professional practice. But the effect on managers in the middle and the staffs they have traditionally managed has yet to be fully appreciated. Some outline features can be discerned:

- The business drive predominates: people take second place to the preservation of the business. Tough decisions are being taken on 'downsizing', ie making employees redundant.

- The middle manager is an endangered species, in the NHS as in other large organisations such as banks. Hierarchies are being 'flattened' with fewer links on the chain of command. For some, this empowers those at the bottom; for others, it increases the workload and stress.

- Employment conditions are becoming less secure and more individualised. There is less protection available from national terms and conditions from the collective action of trades unions and professional associations. Again, for some, a greater individualism and insecurity strikes terror into their hearts; for others, there is a sense of greater liberation and the opening up of opportunity after stifling regulation.

These trends from top to bottom of the organisation suggest that new ways of managing people must be found and managers developed to cope with them. The NHS is already beginning to conform to Handy's 'shamrock' organisation – a tripartite structure consisting of core full time workers, part-time, temporary workers and contract workers (Handy 1989). Each segment requires a different management approach. Flexibility is being demanded from the workforce: flexibility will be necessary in managing its various parts. The 'people' item will rise up the business planning agenda in the remainder of the decade as managers learn how to take more seriously the development of their greatest asset.

Purchaser development

In the run-up to the implementation of the reforms in April 1991, policy-makers' attention was fixed on the establishment of provider mechanisms, especially the NHS trusts. Guy's Hospital, the NHS trust flagship, was rarely off the television screens, and its 'new' Chief Executive came from the post of Deputy Chief Executive at the NHS Management Executive (ME). The replacement Deputy Chief Executive at the ME turned the spotlight on the hitherto neglected purchasing function, which had been glossed over in the White Paper as mainly a matter of agreeing contacts with providers (DoH 1989a).

It soon became apparent that this function was potentially the most innovative in the reformed NHS, and much effort has subsequently gone into understanding it and constructing a new infrastructure. It is from this work that a whole new syllabus for developing managerial skills is emerging.

As a result of research commissioned by the ME, the hallmarks of what makes an effective purchaser have been established. These include: a strategic approach; open and accessible to the public; assessing health need more systematically; obtaining professional advice; involving GPs; working with other agencies; using contracts more effectively; a mature relationship with providers; building structures and skills (Ham, Thompson and Tremblay 1993). Perhaps, sadly, it can be recognised that this agenda is just what senior NHS managers should have been addressing since 1948, or at least 1974. And indeed, they have always given some attention to them. But the reforms have bought a fresh emphasis and intensity.

As is usual with NHS reorganisation, much energy initially goes into new structures and roles, as senior managers secure their personal positions. This has provided an important foundation for approaching new tasks. An interesting variety of infrastructures is appearing around the country, often reflecting the character of the region, from the formalised orderliness of Wessex to the eclecticism of the West Midlands. It will be important to research the success with which key issues have been resolved: purchaser size and mergers, relations between District Health Authority purchasers and Family Health Service Authorities, interface with Local Authorities and other agencies, links with GPs and providers.

This is an area where organisation development and traditional management development blur. Structures tend to evolve from the existing pattern, but the new purchasing authorities are very new institutions, where functions, roles and competencies must be understood before new structures are cemented in place. They are small but powerful, in an NHS more used to equating size with power – size of budget, staff and premises. Purchasing staffs are characterised by being few in number, but more highly specialised and senior in proportion to provider staffing. The process of developing this new organisation is likely to continue for a number of years, perhaps until the end of the decade; if no substantial political upheaval intervenes.

Organisation development in the broad sense needs to be matched by the acquisition of key managerial skills. It has become generally recognised among purchasers that they must be able to assess health need. This has largely become the province of public health medicine specialists, whose annual reports are supplying the building bricks for the purchasing plan. But it is also clear that there is a history of neglect in this area, and that more expertise will be required to impact on the material. Existing specialists are hard pressed often to produce more than a good demographic and epidemiological survey and an analysis of a selected number of conditions or services, such as coronary heart disease or diabetes. They are unlikely to produce a comprehensive picture with existing resources.

Second, the acquisition of such hard information should be matched by the search for softer intelligence. The challenge here is to seek the views of the (taxpaying) public, who have been largely ignored for 45 years. It is pleasing to see a variety of methods being attempted around the country: surveys in-house and by polling firms, public meetings, telephone interviews etc. Managers and their advisors will undoubtedly develop the skills of direct contact quite rapidly where there is a will. But there remains a feeling of dabbling daringly in dangerous waters. Expectations may be aroused which have no hope of being met. Worse, the public may express preferences which do not conform to professional priorities, such as the closure of long stay hospitals. There is a long way to go before managers learn to handle such issues with confidence and credibility. In the meantime, soft intelligence can enrich the purchasing plan: for example, it can reveal whether the public are prepared to travel further to reduce the waiting time for treatment.

A third skill area embraces the processes of establishing a strategic vision, setting priorities and contracting with providers. These require both creative and analytic intellectual effort and a tactical capability. The purchasing plan must be coherent and credible to a greater extent than has been demanded before from senior NHS managers. The capabilities required for producing it have been discovered by purchasers learning by doing. They were not clearly envisaged in the White Paper formulation, which saw only as far as the contracting element. The practical development of managers in these skills is in need of supporting research into the processes involved. It is an area where best practice should be captured and disseminated to other purchasers. The NHS has never been markedly good at learning from its own demonstrations, but there is an urgency about this element of purchasing which demands an unprecedented opening of minds to what is discovered elsewhere.

The final aspect of developing purchasing management is arguably the most crucial: vital even to the success of the White Paper reforms themselves. It is this which will, or will not, distinguish these reforms from previous re-organisations. It is on the purchasers that the burden of creating real change is falling. The challenge is to make a real shift in the historic pattern of the dominance of professionally driven, high technology secondary and tertiary care, which swallows the lion's share of resources to treat a minority of patients. Purchasing managers are contemplating the task of managing change on a scale not seen before. Already there is some interesting work on altering the balance of care within specialties or care groups, eg putting more resources into preventing stroke and less into 'curing' it. The detail of service contracts can enforce this pattern, if soundly monitored. The real challenge will come with proposals for a more fundamental shift in the pattern of care from secondary to primary. The London health care scene is the cauldron for this debate, following the publication of the Tomlinson Report in November 1992 and the Government's calculated response in the face of fierce opposition from the elite medical institutions. This debate is being repeated in microcosm throughout the NHS, and it is at the time of writing unclear whether purchasing managers possess the confidence and competence to secure crucial changes.

The probability is that the task will prove beyond them, as professionals triumph and politicians quail. In this case, no amount of management development will save the NHS from contemplating still further reforms. These will be characterised by further attempts to put public before provider, and health care before cure. Politicians may at last realise that this can never be achieved by slicing away at hospital services and giving the pieces to primary care. The place to start is primary care: the foundation on which the rest may be built.

Involving doctors in management

The continuing saga of attempts to involve clinicians in management is a refrain reverberating through both provider and purchaser development. Overt attempts to involve clinicians date back at least to the Cogwheel Reports of 1967–69. It was a central plank of the Griffiths recommendations of 1983 and the evidence suggests that success was only fitful and scattered (Hunter and Williamson 1989). It is probably still the greatest challenge facing management developers – and others, of course – in the 1990s, and as such will be examined in more detail here.

The case for clinician involvement has been rehearsed many times and is taken as already established. The fundamental problem appears to lie in the balance of power within the NHS as an organisation. Clinicians have been accustomed to having the prime influence over the deployment of resources and to enjoying considerable freedom to pursue their professional activities. As agents of government, managers have been gradually given more 'structural' power to control the 'expert' power of the professional. Among wise men and women, there is a respect for the contribution of clinicians and managers. Among the unlucky and the foolish, there is the potential for damaging conflict.

The question of the balance of power will be debated and decided at a political level. This focus of controversy has underpinned the implementation of the White Paper. For managers, the issue manifested itself initially at a more procedural level, revolving around resource management. This issue was the subject of the previous chapter and will not be discussed here, except to identify the implications for management development.

These turn, in part, on a conceptual question: who are the managers? To what extent are the managers those with an identifiable managerial responsibility, such as general managers, senior managers and indeed clinical directors? Or are they all those who 'manage' resources, which must include all senior clinicians. It would seem only prudent and realistic to adopt the wider definition, otherwise the management developer risks ignoring substantial numbers of powerful people who 'make things happen' in health care. The management developer must now contemplate two powerful groups of clinicians in management. One group is familiar, the other is rather newer.

The familiar group – a rose by another name – consists of clinical directors. These now carry the traditional burden of the senior hospital doctor in management. As officially envisaged, they emerge as powerful managerial functionaries: line managers, deployers of a wide range of medical, nursing and supporting resources, purchasers of other services, able to influence policy. In practice, they have found it difficult to live up to these managerial expectations while maintaining a considerable clinical practice. They have usually not enjoyed much development for these demanding managerial roles and the time they can devote is strictly limited: two sessions a week and as much spare time as they can stand. The result for many has been disillusionment and compromise. Some have been shifted *de facto* or even *de jure* from line responsibility which is assumed by their business manager and sometimes their senior nurse: their title becomes 'clinical co-ordinator'. Many have not been able to establish managerial authority over their clinical colleagues; some have given up even trying.

As in all aspects of an organisation as big as the NHS, good practice can be found: there are examples of successful clinical directors. But there are too many NHS trusts which have not implemented the approach soundly. The result is a hole at the centre of the management structure: a discontinuity between higher management and service deliverers. This suggests a massive need for organisational and manager development. Structures need to be reviewed and made credible; managers, including the clinical directors, require both individual and team development. All too often, both types of development have been squeezed out by day to day priorities and crises.

Many NHS Trust chief executives report a tension with their clinical directors, a lack of support in achieving the business plan. Many clinical directors complain of being kept in the dark, of being denied in practice what freedoms they were initially promised. This lack of mutual confidence, sufficiently widespread, is a major problem of development.

The second group of clinicians to enter the wider management arena is new: the GP fundholders. They constitute arguably the most exciting newcomers to arise from the purchaser–provider split. They are worthy of attention from management developers, because it is from them that real change may come: the aggregate of many small improvements which GP funds may purchase. Like gravel thrown into a pond, the ripples of many small purchasing decisions will not create a big wave, but will nonetheless lap on many shores. An active and well-organised GP fundholding practice with real money to spend can force new responsiveness on their local provider hospitals. The doors of once supercilious consultants are now open. It can also create a stir in the traditional NHS bureaucracies, not yet wedded to the entrepreneurial culture. Officials at region, at district purchasing, at FHSA, cry 'accountability' and argue for greater integration of fundholders in 'strategic' purchasing plans. This is logical and reasonable. But it was George Bernard Shaw who said in 1910 that 'all progress depends on the unreasonable man'.

In this light, the NHS should preserve and develop its GP fund-holders. Each fundholding practice can give examples of real health gain for individual patients which could not have been secured without the availability of real and ready money. The impression given by a brief survey of first wave fundholders (Ham, Honigsbaum and Thompson 1993) suggests that they were among the most able and organised of GP practices: close to their patients, up to date with best clinical practice, on top of their information requirements, and well financed. They hold many lessons for management developers who may soon be faced with later waves of fundholders, or even non-fundholders, who will be in need of development. This is a highly fragmented field of development, but one which is important to cultivate in the interest of change and real health gain.

The infrastructure issue

In the new world of purchasers and providers, there are clearly several great development tasks to be addressed. What are the implications for management development infrastructure and roles? The first edition of this book noted the tensions inherent in the balance between centralised and localised infrastructure. Since the early days of management development in the NHS, in the 1960s, there were always valuable initiatives at the centre and in localities. Activities were, as always in NHS management, varied as to geographical spread and personal commitment but, in the main, there was a clear division between local effort for local benefit, and central sponsorship for the general good. For example, NHS National Education Centres offered general development programmes at middle and senior levels for which any suitable manager could be nominated. Junior and first line managers tended to be provided for locally by Health Authority specialists and/or local colleges.

The advent of the NHS Training Authority in 1985 gave a great boost to management development nationally. The publication of the review report *Better Management, Better Health* (BM, BH) in 1986 was an occasion of great significance. It constituted the first comprehensive review of management development since the mid-1970s, and the first time that management development requirements were discussed nationally in the context of an explicit notion of 'management'. The major achievement of BM, BH was to move 'development' closer to the central concerns of 'management', and away from the province of the management development specialist. This was asserted in its definition of management development as:

> *any influence or experience that helps to improve managerial effectiveness.*
> *(NHS Training Authority 1986)*

Additionally, each Health Authority had to identify a local person with responsibility for implementing management development strategies. Stimulated by this policy initiative and other favourable encouragement, there was an apparent upsurge in development activity. New programmes were launched nationally: Individual Performance Review, National Accelerated Development Programme etc. The enduring problem of preparing clinicians to participate in management was tackled. It was estimated that more than half the 200 Health Authorities in England and Wales designated a responsible officer, and that there was a greater volume and variety of activity than ever before: traditional courses were supplemented by a new range of imaginative options, to which more managers than ever before had access (Thompson and Edmonstone 1988).

There was, however, a serious contradiction in the Training Authority's approach. In keeping with the emerging philosophy of the NHS, there was a concern to obtain better value for money by encouraging a 'market' among management development suppliers. From September 1987, the traditional 'block grants' to a cartel of National Education Centres were withdrawn and the market was thrown open to any suppliers to compete for contracts. At national level, the training Authority could thus ensure that its contracts were led to suppliers who would work to tightly drawn specifications. Locally, Health Authorities were encouraged to buy what specialist management development they felt fitted their needs, and to meet the full cost of their requirements. Programmes would wither away if they did not command sufficient local support.

The essential contradiction lay in the incompatibilities of 'command' policies and 'market' practice. Nationally endorsed policies suggest a need for consistency and co-ordination in implementation. Consistency is difficult to achieve if the policies are in competition with other priorities at local level. In practice, management development proposals find it hard to claim managers' interest in the face of demand for improved patient care, professional training etc. So the manager or 'customer' may choose not to buy on this occasion.

At the supplier end, education providers were encouraged to behave commercially, with the penalty coming from lack of co-ordination. They have naturally sought competitive advantage and been reluctant to share their experience and expertise with their 'rivals'. With prices honed to the bone, very little surplus has been available for ensuring a solid infrastructure and the means of continuity.

A central organ such as the Training Authority naturally found it difficult to relax its hold completely but, unless it can 'command' the situation, it falls to the mercies of local 'market' economies. A notable example of this occurred when the Authority attempted to implement a process of 'accrediting' management centres and 'recognising' Health Authorities who met appropriate standards. In 1987 a working party produced a very worthy report for the Training Authority outlining a six-step process involving self-appraisal, a review team visit and adjudication by an accreditation/recognition panel. This scheme found no favour with either purchasers or providers of management development. The process was seen to be too cumbersome and costly to provide much useful guidance to purchasers, who, in any case, preferred to back their own judgement. Providers felt that a good 'product' or service would be bought with, or without, the Training Authority's stamp of approval.

Unless the Training Authority backed its proposals with hard cash, it found itself drawn increasingly into the market in a rather ambiguous purchase/supplier role. A further and more complex instance of this was the National Accelerated Development Programme (NADP). The merits of the programme itself are debated below, but in spite of considerable resources expended, the programme never took on its comprehensive scope. While many of the components came into existence, they were never co-ordinated into a proper national programme. Thus the NADP became synonymous with three General Management Development Schemes (GMTS) and never deployed the full range of intended option, especially the use of 'designated posts'. The processes of Individual Performance Review and Personal Development Planning functioned only fitfully, and were distorted by their association with Performance Related Pay. While many individuals gained from GMTS programmes, others were inhibited by the inexperienced use of assessment centres to identify 'fast track' potential. The national impetus became diffused into regional effort, with consequent fragmentation and inconsistency of standards.

At the other end of the managerial hierarchy was the ambitious Management Education Syllabus and Open Learning (MESOL) project sponsored by the Training Authority and devised by the Open University and the Institute of Health Service Management. Later entitled Managing Health Services, the aim was to invest in a distance learning system and materials appropriate for some 70,000 NHS managers at the threshold of their managerial careers, with a take up of 3,000 participants per year, at a cost somewhere between £100,000 to £300,000 for initial development. The Training Authority controlled the development of system and materials through direct funding but it had to be marketed to the NHS in competition with a multitude of alternatives, many of which were long established and closely adapted to local needs. It was not easy but it succeeded because it suited the market, rather than because it was implemented as national policy.

The review in the first edition of this book pointed to the confusion in the Training Authority's role: either it had to be strengthened as an effective arm of central policy, or it should be abolished so that the market – created by itself – could have free play. In the intervening two years, the market has won. In April 1991, the Authority was replaced by a Training Directorate under the control of the NHS Director of Personnel.

A 'demand-led' strategy?

In spite of the abolition of the NHS Training Authority, there is a continuing need for policy guidance for development from the centre. At the very minimum, the NHS Management Executive needs the availability of skilled advice. The source of this advice is an indicator of the cultural shift in the NHS: the advice is now tendered through a single expert of directorial status on the Executive – a 'general management' culture – not collectively by an Authority in the traditional manner – a 'consensus' culture.

One policy issue will dominate the middle 1990s: a focus on what might be called 'competition policy'. It will be necessary to decide on the amount of resource to invest in management development, and what mechanism should be used to allocate these resources. At present, the reins of central control in management development have been slackened, and provider units and NHS trusts – where most managers are found – have been freer to decide for themselves. This has faced management development proposals with hard competition from patient care, business and professional imperatives. The generalised and longer-term values of the former are always likely to be seen to a disadvantage against the more immediate and more publicly 'acceptable' benefits of the latter.

It is for the Management Executive to consider the merits of investment in NHS managers and, as necessary, to ease the competitive situation locally. The temptation is to establish a structure which relies on the initiatives of experts – Training Directorate, Regional Training Departments, Management Development Advisers. This was one of the messages in the White Paper Working Paper 10 concerning Education and Training (DoH 1989b). This largely constitutes the road that the NHS Training Directorate has gone down in the two years of its existence so far. It has become a major commissioner and indeed supplier itself of training 'products'. This has served to confuse its role in the purchaser–provider world, and has sometimes diminished the impact of its valuable policy statements.

Thus its Management Development Strategy for the NHS, published in October 1991, was an insightful and progressive document. It summarised substantial research into the current and planned provision of management development in the changing NHS and clearly set out national policy in terms of the Management Executive's values and expectation (NHS Training Directorate 1991). It is in the action plan that the weaknesses become apparent. The plan assumes a unitary organisation in which national and regional levels 'support' the local implementation of the strategy. This world has now disappeared as the timescale for the eight key measures clearly demonstrates. All the target dates have now passed with very little achieved, except perhaps some practices which are a little more 'woman friendly'. Even the establishment of a national management centre does not seem to have survived its principal sponsors. All this seems to endorse the history of the 1970s and 1980s which suggested that a 'supply-led' strategy would have a very limited success.

An alternative – and theoretically the more sound approach – is a 'demand-led' strategy in which chief executives and general managers are committed to investment in development because they can see its importance to the achievement of the business plan. Given their commitment, resources will be found and expertise deployed where it is wanted by them and not where remote policy makers of self-interested specialists would prefer.

To what extent is this a threat to the management development specialist? In the short term, it may upset established practices. But, in the longer term, it promises to move the specialist closer to the levers of power, which have often eluded his or her grasp, leaving a sense of being on the periphery of events.

Nor need specialists be passive spectators during any transition in strategy. They can and should influence events. One of the challenges is to engage more convincingly in the process of evaluation, especially in relation to the business plan. This has always constituted something of an Achilles Heel: it has been impossible to prove the value of development activity in most cases. It remains an act of common sense or even faith. The problems of evaluation are well known, and a number of approaches are available in the writing of Easterby-Smith and others (Easterby-Smith 1981). The task for the NHS developer is to be more careful in evaluating learning and to make the findings more visible to policy-makers.

A weakness of the comprehensive review in *Better Management, Better Health* was that it did not make explicit the value of development activities. The important Part 1 of the report demonstrated the need for development with admirable clarity, but there was no 'bridge' to the recommendations on good practices. It was assumed that they would meet the need. In future, management developers are going to have to make the connection much clearer, and the evidence of evaluation will be vital.

Formal and informal development approaches

The 1970s and 1980s witnessed a striking growth in the range of development options available to NHS managers. The traditional short, off-the-job course, first used in the mid-1960s, became a flexible and sophisticated tool, joined by a host of less formalised techniques.

In the later 1980s, the predominance of the short, 'continuing education' event gave way to a polarisation between formal 'educational' programmes, such as Certificates in Management Studies and MBAs, and informal work-place, problem-solving learning, often associated with consultancy. The former approach offers the student a continuity of learning, although often within an academic rather than a practical framework. The value of the latter often comes from relevance to managerial concerns, but its immediacy can often drive out its usefulness as a source of learning.

Between the mid-1960s and mid-1980s, there was a range of centrally funded short development courses available on a national basis to eligible managers from all disciplines at middle and senior levels. They were sponsored successively by the DHSS, NHS National Training Council and NHS Training Authority. The latter body intended that the programmes should become self-financing, but the National Education Centres who were the major providers found that employers were not attracted by full-cost funding.

At best, these courses integrated the twin goals of relevance and continuity by providing a set of learning experiences over 4–6 months which enable several thousand NHS managers to have their first and, in many cases, only systematic opportunity of development.

With the almost total demise of these courses, the running has been taken up by the education sector with an increasingly comprehensive variety of accredited programmes. Academic barriers to learning in the form of 'gateway' qualifications have been progressively diminished until even the most hidebound institution have evolved 'open-access' programmes. Recent evidence suggest that more NHS managers than ever before are studying by one mode or another for certificates, diplomas, graduate degrees and postgraduate degrees in relevant managerial subjects. Since many of these are financed by their NHS employers, there is at least *prima facie* evidence that these employers will be looking for outcomes in terms of enhanced performance.

At the informal end of the spectrum, learning opportunities have crept even nearer to the workplace. All too often, however, progress depends on the energy of individual managers and the support of their superiors. Techniques such as Individual Performance Review and Personal Development Plans have helped, but will not guarantee any action. But, just as there is less and less surprise at managers studying for masters and doctoral qualifications, there is equally diminishing resistance to informal learning events involving learning sets, time out reviews, even one-to-one coaching.

Perhaps the demand for high-calibre and competent managers throughout the 1990s will guarantee the continuation of this 'twin-track' strategy of formal and informal development, guided by policies and monitoring from the centre. There is, however, a strong case to be made for the retention of management development expertise available to the NHS. Much of the 'provision' can be, and is being, bought in from independent or semi-independent contractors. But there is a need to ensure a capacity for expert advice which will depend on the continuous involvement of experts with the complexities and problems of the NHS. There is a central role for specialists who can integrate the formal with informal, who are able to influence the centres of power, and are committed more closely to the mission of the NHS than just financial reward.

References

Department of Health 1989a *Working for Patients* The White Paper HMSO, London

Department of Health 1989b *Education and Training* Working Paper 10 HMSO, London

Department of Health and Social Security 1983 *NHS Management Inquiry* The Griffiths Report DHSS, London

Easterby-Smith M 1981 'The evaluation of management education and development: an overview' *Personnel Review* 10(2)

Ham C, Honigsbaum F and Thompson D 1993 *Priority Setting for Health Gain*. The University of Birmingham, HSMC unpublished report, Birmingham

Ham C, Thompson D and Tremblay M 1993 *Effective Purchasing*. The University of Birmingham, HSMC unpublished report, Birmingham

Handy C 1989 *The Age of Unreason*. Business Books Ltd, London

Hunter D and Williamson P (eds) 1989 'Perspectives on general management in the NHS' *Health Services Management Research* **2**, 1

Kotler P 1988 *Marketing Management Analysis, Planning, Implementation and Control*. Prentice Hall, Englewood Cliffs, New Jersey

Le Grand J 1990 *Quasi Markets and Social Policy*. SAUS Publications, University of Bristol, Bristol

NHS Training Authority 1986 *Better Management, Better Health* NHS Training Authority, Bristol

NHS Training Directorate 1991 *A Management Development Strategy for the NHS* NHS Training Directorate, Bristol

Thompson D and Edmonstone J 1988 *Resources for Management Development* NHS Training Authority, Bristol

Williams D 1988 'Have we achieved better management, better health?' *Health Services Manpower Review* March

7 Managing the human resources of the NHS in the 1990s

Hugh Flanagan

The foundations of organisational success

During the 1980s most writers and researchers concluded that there were four key components of the culture of successful companies. These were:

- first, a clearly articulated and understood mission or vision which clarified the purpose of the organisation;

- second a coherent strategy for its achievement;

- third, both the first two must be clearly and consistently communicated to the people who are going to make it happen;

- fourth, all three must be built on and reflect a set of values that make people feel important to and respected by the organisation.

Most of these ideas stem from what has now come to be known as the 'excellence' literature, much of which started with the work of McKinseys and Peters and Watermann. Successful companies are 'people orientated', treat 'workers as the most important asset', like 'grown-ups' and show 'respect for the individual'. (Peters and Watermann 1982) 'The companies with reputations for progressive human resource practices were significantly higher in long-term profitability and financial growth than their counterparts'. (Kanter 1984) 'Values and beliefs cannot be created out of thin air. Unless they are real, and permeate everything that is done, they will not have any effect'. (Harvey-Jones 1988)

There was a clear message from all the studies of, and in all the literature on 'excellence' which emphasised the strategic importance of the people in the organisation – its human resource – and their key role in achieving strategic goals and the delivery of a high quality service. It is a message with which we are now all familiar but is it yet operationalised in any meaningful or useful way? What difference has it made to the NHS? 'The frequently heard cliche that "people are our most important asset" still rings hollow in many organisations'. (Buller 1988)

From the middle of the 1980s new terminology began to appear of which three principal examples are that of 'quality' – Crosby, Deeming Oakwood etc – which though not new assumed a prominence during the 1980s right across public and private sector organisation and more lately that of 'performance management' which does not yet have gurus of the prominence of Deeming *et al.* and the learning organisation or the flexible firm (Sange 1990, Garrett 1987). Although these 'new' ideas put a different slant on the approach to organisational success or excellence an examination of the literature, research and case studies of good practice continue to support and indeed emphasize the importance of the four factors referred to above and all they imply and add a fifth component – adaptability.

• The capacity of organisations to continually examine the internal process, systems and structures to ensure maximum performance in current circumstances, whilst at the same time scanning their external environment to identify factors which may affect their future survival and success and setting in train internal changes at a rate which matches and preferably exceeds the changes in the environment.

Unfortunately there are still far too many examples both in the public and private sectors of organisations and senior managers where consideration or discussion of these basic requirements creates either embarrassment, cynicism or a feeling of helplessness. The new NHS organisations are not exempted, for example, many organisations now have mission statements but no sense of mission. Nicely presented and often carefully worded mission statements are issued by 'the board' on the assumption that this is all that is needed and that staff will understand and automatically subscribe to their content, without the level of communication and participative discussion needed to give meaning to a set of words. It is the process of producing the words that is of value to the organisation. A similar point can be made about quality statements and initiatives and the introduction of performance management systems which are not either understood by a sufficient majority of people in the organisation – a critical mass – or integrated with other systems and processes as part of a coherent strategy. The result is often more cynicism and greater stress.

The change in beliefs and behaviour required to achieve an involving process seems to be considerably more than many organisations, including health service organisations, are able to manage. Is this due mainly to a fundamentally opposite set of beliefs about managing people on the part of managers, a lack of competence when faced with the complexities of managing people or an environment that doesn't encourage and may even positively discourage such an approach?

Combining a performance orientation with a real concern for people is a difficult balancing act but some organisations do manage it.

Organisations may espouse certain ideas, but do nothing practical, or, may do something but in a way that ignores the core purpose for which the organisation exists. In other words, they don't combine a performance orientation with respect for the individual and the approach is not consistent and holistic. Treating people well because it is the right and civilised thing to do, must in the context of an organisation be linked to whatever the core purpose of that organisation is. At the same time, appearing to treat people well solely because we know we can get more out of them will not be sufficient to achieve high performance in the long-term. It will rightly be viewed as manipulation. Doing one thing, because it is expedient, but believing another, will inevitably reveal itself in a whole host of ways to those who are 'being done to'.

'Policies about people must inevitably express values, assumptions and the received wisdom of management about how to motivate, and to create harmonious relationships'. (Tyson and Fell 1986) Organisations have to say what they believe, believe what they say and then act on their beliefs. People within the organisation, and those to whom the organisation provides its services, on whom it depends for its survival in a free market, will, anyway, form impressions of the organisations implicit value system from the way it deals with them as employee or customer and respond accordingly.

'Values are beliefs that guide managerial conduct. In the NHS the managerial culture of the service is less clear and confident than it is in the best industrial organisations'. (National Health Service Training Authority 1985) The NHS is (some might say was) an organisation derived – through the mechanism of socialism – from the biblical notion that 'I am my brother's keeper'. Therefore, one should be able to assume that the NHS comes ready made with a set of values that are centred on 'caring' and 'respect' for the individual. However, whilst there are numerous examples from all groups of staff (including managers) of people who care deeply about how patients and staff are treated, there are also many signs and symbols around that signal a lack of concern or care for the individual – whether patient or staff.

Drucker (1990) says something similar in his book on managing the non-profit organisation: 'People don't just work for a living, they work for a cause (at least a good many do). This creates a tremendous responsibility for the organisation 'to keep the flame alive, not to allow work to become just a job'. But, hospitals often seem to 'do the poorest job of keeping that spirit alive'.

Several commentators state that organisational culture can both be identified in and shared through the symbolic forms and the mundane tools of senior management (Gowler and Legge 1986), ie the patterns of actual behaviour of managers and all other staff. The key factor is the actual rather than the espoused approach of the senior managers and professional staff.

Part of the difficulty of manifesting, rather than just espousing a real people orientation so that staff are not just units of production, is the very nature of the NHS. There are clear differences between public and private sector organisations (Stewart and Ranson 1988) and there are problems with defining the nature and purpose of the NHS. (Klein 1982) The commitment of managers in the NHS to a people-orientated set of values is not sufficient, there must be unequivocal political support as well. That seems to be unlikely whatever government is in power because political priorities and timescales do not take account of individual employee needs and what is currently known about managing change. Cost, always a major consideration, is becoming an even more critical driving force.

Other organisations have achieved great success by taking a different approach. The essential difference is that their approach is based on a coherent philosophy of management which provides both a value base and a framework for the organisations' personnel policies. In NHS organisations, personnel policies tend to exist in isolation with minimal relationship to each other, let alone any corporate or strategic plan that might exist.

The NHS increasingly reflects the general concern of the Western approach to management in defining objectives and outcomes. There is nothing intrinsically wrong in this provided it doesn't lead to an overbalanced emphasis on 'the bottom line', and the view that nothing is important unless it can be quantified and involves people in hard tasks. But there is the real danger that such a drive blinds those involved to the broader and deeper realities and dynamics of the situation in which managers are trying to manage. Frequently one hears senior managers discussing the need to 'change attitudes', 'get a greater commitment', get managers to be more performance oriented etc, but there is no evidence of the same managers giving time and energy to action that will enable them to develop an insight into the factors that influence such changes.

Harvey-Jones in his book *Making it Happen* discussed the future success of firms in terms of their ability and preparedness to meet people's needs in the provision of work. 'Increasingly, companies will only survive if they meet the needs of the individuals who serve in them; not just the question of payment, important as this may be, but people's true inner needs which they may even be reluctant to express themselves'. (Harvey-Jones 1988) In the book accompanying his second TV series he describes management as being about continuous change, 'the continuous growth of people and the continuous creation of a better tomorrow out of today . . . it is about gaining the commitment of all the people in the organisation to achievements which they and their customers believe to be better than before'. (Harvey-Jones 1992) He talks about his admiration for the Japanese approach to management because they are continually looking for ways to improve not only the product but also the process by which people work together to make it.

Goldsmith and Clutterbuck in their book *The Winning Streak*, identified eight common characteristics found among successful firms.

They also looked at unsuccessful companies to check out whether or not such organisations also displayed some or all of the characteristics of the successful firms. 'The upshot is that the unsuccessful firms all demonstrated a lack of some or most of the characteristics of success . . . . Those that were still on the downward path appeared to be paying little or no attention to several of these areas'. (Goldsmith and Clutterbuck 1984) The words used by Goldsmith and Clutterbuck to describe the eight characteristics are Leadership, Autonomy, Control, Involvement, Marketing Orientation, Innovation and Integrity. Reading through their detailed descriptions of what these characteristics involve in practice, in terms of what the successful organisations actually *do* and how they are managed, there are clear reflections of the people philosophy and values embodied in all of the 'search for excellence' literature and in much of the work on quality and performance management. There is a consistent and enduring message.

Clutterbuck's later study *The Decline and Rise of British Industry* combined perceptions and quantifiable data and provided a number of recurrent themes which although derived from private sector organisations are as relevant for NHS organisations required to be more business like. For example in their action list for industry, government and other institutions they state the need to invest continuously in all key resources and particularly in people, technology and advanced equipment, at least 10 per cent of sales turnover in training, equipment and product development, and the need to constantly seek ways to increase involvement of the people in the organisation at all levels and to plan for the long term. On the latter point they also urge government to take a long-term planning perspective which is a particularly important point for public sector organisations.

The NHS as a 'good employer'

The values of the society in which an organisation exists are inevitably reflected in that organisation. However the 1990s have attracted the label 'caring' and the notion of community (to replace the defunct concept of society?) has been introduced. During the 1980s, the values that created the notion of the state caring for the individual, whether as a recipient of services or an employee were systematically eroded. Individuals must survive within the 'market'.

Up until 1979 the role of the state as a model employer had for the previous 60 years or so been largely unquestioned. All governments generally 'sought to set a good example to the private sector by encouraging trade union organisation, supporting collective bargaining and offering a high degree of job security'. (Fredman and Maurice 1989) The introduction of Whitley to the NHS in 1948 was an example of this. 'Thatcherism' radically transformed this position by emphasizing the primacy of the market. National bargaining systems have been restricted if not dismantled and scope for industrial action by trades unions has been limited. 'The Thatcher Government sees trades unions as an unjustifiable interference in the operation of the market, an obstacle to efficiency and incompatible to individual freedom'. (Fredman and Maurice 1989) Job security in the public sector is no greater than in private sector organisations. It is arguable whether the terms and conditions for many staff are now comparatively as good. Low pay continues to be a major social issue.

In most respects the traditional model of the state as an employer is in direct conflict with the values embodied in the free market which was and largely still is seen as the most efficient way to organise the delivery of services. Central to what was referred to as 'Thatcherism' was the idea that the role of the state in the provision of services should be reduced to a minimum, which called into question the very nature of the idea of public service employment. Contracting out, competitive tendering and the 'privatisation' of many services formally provided by the civil service or local authorities together with the introduction of the internal market within the National Health Service have made some fundamental changes not only to the way services are delivered but the employment relationship with 'public servants'.

The continuance of the Whitley Council system throughout the 1990s is questionable, though there is a central inertia which counterbalances any local radicalism. Local pay flexibility in relation to geography, skill and performance have become established principles, though not extensive practice. It was assumed that local flexibility in respect of pay and conditions and other linked working practices would be given an impetus because of the problems of recruitment and retention brought on by the demographic changes. But the continuation of the recession beyond expected timescales largely masked the effect of this; though 'pay and reward' as an issue is still on the agenda but perhaps for slightly different reasons and perceived in a slightly different way. Self governing Trusts acting as autonomous employers being free to determine their own terms and conditions of service, without reference to national agreements is not yet fully a reality and in some cases is proving to be less attractive and more problematic than at first anticipated. The existing Whitley rates and terms of conditions still provide a much needed point of reference. Local radicalism is not yet much in evidence. Whatever the national situation either in terms of Whitley or the local/national labour market there will be a continuing tendency toward some 'mechanism' which will seek to establish a local or regional baseline if only to avoid the obvious problem of wage spirals and leapfrogging within a cash limited NHS.

The restrictions of legislation and creation of smaller independent employing Units has meant that in terms of industrial action, the scope of trades unions is considerably limited in that they are expected to confine any industrial action to the particular unit in question. However this issue has not yet really been tested.

Another consequence of the market philosophy in employment is to introduce a much wider range of flexible working practices than has been the case in the civil service. (Management and Personnel Office 1987) Some of these examples such as increased part-time working (even for senior managers), home-working, seasonal-working, ie with holidays off, are already being considered by a number of Trusts. These are all practices which are characterised by a greater degree of employment insecurity which might be seen as mechanisms for reducing the cost of labour. Many of these arrangements are more suited to married women who also wish to be able to devote time and energy to their families, thus increasing the proportion of part-time female staff in relation to full-time male employees.

The guiding role of the state as a good employer has clearly changed. There was a shift of some sort in the attitudes and values of our society during the 1980s which has affected organisational values and employment practices. The influence of the European Community (in spite of resistance to the social chapter?) will continue to affect the nature of the relationship between those who employ and those who are employed. The philosophy of deregulation and labour market flexibility runs counter to the European Community's philosophy that basic employment rights and standards should be guaranteed and not undermined by increasing competition resulting from the post-1992 European Community market. Countries such as West Germany with higher labour standards have the most to lose if there is not a uniform approach because firms may relocate in areas with less regulation of, and lower standards in, employment rights, eg the UK? In the public sector, it is possible that this could result in a net flow of skilled staff to those countries that offer at least initially, the best relative salary levels and conditions of employment, ie those with higher employment standards, though these would not be the only variables in the situation. At the same time, in the same countries, there might be increased competition from redundant employees in the private sector due to firms relocating to less-regulated countries thus producing a short-term glut of labour in the public sector. In the longer term, any reduction in the economic viability of a country will ultimately affect the salaries and conditions in the public sector and probably result in a net outflow. We have already seen examples of firms moving from Great Britain to France and vice versa and it will take some years for the effects of European employment legislation and other inter-related factors to become clear.

To what extent will community legislation supersede national legislation and interests? An area of major uncertainty is the issue of participation and consultation of workers, a fundamental and recurring theme in community social policy which has been strongly opposed by Britain. In the area of collective bargaining and trade union membership, community proposals to guarantee rights have also been strongly opposed. Proposals on maximum working hours, minimum holidays and the rights of part-time workers provoke British opposition. The ultimate effect of these, and other proposals, on the employment relationship either in terms of legal requirements and of changing expectations on the part of staff is uncertain. That there will be some effect is clear. The NHS, as probably the major employer in Europe, cannot but be affected in terms of its approach to managing its human resources whether in terms of the salaries and wages and terms and conditions of services it offers its staff, its approach to recruiting and retaining the skills it needs, and the nature of the relationship it has with its employees and their representative organisations. To compete for what may be increasingly mobile skills and mobile employees it will have to seek to be among the best in Europe and to be people centred. This will not only mean being reasonably competitive in terms of what it pays its staff, but probably more importantly that its staff really do believe that 'the NHS' and specifically the organisations that directly employ them do see them as the most important asset. This message will have to be clearly communicated and made manifest in all interactions with staff. The problem, in part, will be identifying what 'the NHS' is – who ultimately influences and fixes the values that underpin the NHS approach to managing its people? Is it the political masters of the system or the managers of the system? Can Trusts really get it right because they have greater control? Will their top managers have the final say, in the way an independent company in the private sector can? Even then, to what extent will they be controlled by European and National legislation and influenced by the internal systems and processes of the NHS?

The mid-1990s show signs of rising job losses in the public sector. Although there will always be a demand for health care workers, the economic situation both because of its direct impact on PSBR (irrespective of gradual improvement) and the general philosophy of efficiency and cost minimization it has engendered, is building greater pressure to reduce the cost of labour in health organisations. The effect of this could be to cause senior managers to deal with people as a 'factor of production', a cost to be held down, which will drive the approach to managing people in the NHS. This in turn would be likely to result in reduced commitment, flexibility and integration and destructive rather constructive conflict – a return to the 'dark ages' of the 1970s? Hopefully anticipation of this scenario will avoid its worst possibilities.

From personnel management to human resource management

Key to much of what happens will be the approach to the management of people generally adopted within the NHS. This section looks at the development of the personnel function and the personnel department. Personnel officers began to appear in the NHS in the late 1960s and early 1970s. The 1974 reorganisation firmly established the role of area and district personnel officers in the structure and hierarchy of the NHS. The personnel function developed and established itself throughout the 1970s mainly in response to the problems of industrial action and increasing trade unionisation within the National Health Service and the background of new employment legislation. It could be said to have brought about post Donovan proceduralism in the NHS, ie the formalisation of rules, agreements and relationships between administration (or management) and the TUs. (Donovan 1968) At the risk of over generalising, the personnel role up to the early 1980s could be described as 'conflict containment and resolution together with the administration of various personnel activities'. During the 1980s the personnel function assumed a much greater role in the management of change, and increasingly has been expected to take on a wider remit with extended corporate responsibilities. In the 1990s the language is all about 'business driven HRM'.

Human Resource Management (HRM) is seen as something different to, and something more than, 'traditional' personnel management, ie an attempt to manage productively and more systematically in line with overall business strategy the people resources of the organisation from recruitment through to retirement. Human Resource Management is primarily concerned with organising the people in the organisation in a way that is most beneficial to the achievement of the organisations purpose. Deliberate use of the term 'human resource management' should indicate a very different philosophy of management to that implied by the term 'personnel management'.

It is easy to be cynical, and sometimes rightly so, about changes in title which describe the work of a particular function or specialty in management. Often such semantic changes illustrate aspiration rather than reality. But, there are an increasing number of significant examples of change in the way that organisations are managing the relationship with their employees.

Many 'personnel' departments are trying to take a radical look at their purpose, relationships and methods of working. Is its purpose to be conflict containing and resolving and status quo orientated, or is it to be the conscience of the organisation? Should its purpose be to contribute in a much more fundamental way to the nature and purpose of the 'business'? Is its role to influence and to facilitate a clear understanding and articulation of the 'mission' of the organisation to all involved in its achievement, contributing both to the formulation of corporate strategies as well as their implementation? The answer is that it is all of these and more in different mixes for different organisational situations.

Torrington (1988) discusses a number of assumptions he makes differentiating between 'personnel management' and 'human resources management'. Personnel management is focussed on the employees in the organisation in terms of recruiting and training them, arranging for them to be paid, agreeing on the nature of the contract of employment within collective agreements, explaining (hopefully) what is expected of them, and justifying what management is doing or attempting to do and seeking to modify that action where it could produce conflict with employee interests. A pluralist view of the organisation prevails. The theory, and to a larger extent the practice, of personnel management is concerned with understanding employee attitudes, interests and responses not only because it is a 'good thing' to do so but because of the need to obtain the commitment and cooperation of employees and to minimise their *cost* to the organisation, in order for it to succeed. Labour is seen as a factor of production. This often places the personnel manager in some kind of mediator role between employees and managers because of the need for someone in the organisation to have a more detailed understanding of the views, attitudes and expectations of the employees, why they hold them, and to be able to articulate these views to and within the management function of the organisation.

The focus of human resource management is quite different. Instead of starting with the workforce as given, in terms of the available skills, numbers, attitudes etc, and as representing a cost to the organisation, human resource management starts from the point of *need* for human resources by the organisation. People are the resource through which the inanimate factors of production are turned into wealth. This is a focus on the demand side rather than on the supply side. It plays down mediation and adopts a unitary perspective. There is a strong emphasis on direction and the development of strategies to achieve that direction rather than on solving problems in relation to the interface between employer and employee. The essential need for employee cooperation 'is delivered by programmes of corporate culture, remuneration packaging, team building and management development for core employees, while peripheral employees are kept at arms length'. (Torrington 1988) There are already many examples both in the public and private sector of the core and periphery workforce concept, eg contracting out which is far more widespread than might at first be assumed. Most people in the NHS will think of 'contracting out' in terms of the traditional ancillary services but in fact there is a much wider spread of contracting arrangements across a whole range of services, including 'personnel' or 'human resourcing' services.

The unitary perspective embodied within the concept of human resource management could be argued to be an outcome of the value set that developed during the 1980s in the UK, manifested in the governments attitude to trades unions. There is generally less room for diverging views and within the health service one can identify a number of examples where a pluralist perspective is no longer so acceptable, not only with regard to the traditional trades unions but in terms of the tolerance for the professionals to operate on the basis of attitudes or aspirations different from those being promulgated both explicitly and implicitly from the top of the organisation.

Within the health service the more responsibility a Trust has for itself and its success then the treater will be the need for all those involved in the delivery of its services to patients to have a unitary perspective on the importance of the delivery of those services, their method of delivery and to be committed in a very practical way to the achievement of a high quality, low cost service defined by any contractual agreement governing the provision of the services.

These differences between personnel management and human resource management have now merged into the debate about 'hard' and 'soft' HRM which is largely American in origin. The hard approach focusses on the 'resource' idea. People should be managed like any other resource, purchased as cheaply as possible and used frugally taking into account the need for quality and efficiency. They should be developed and exploited as fully and profitably as possible. Sub-contracting and other manifestations of the core-periphery idea are entirely appropriate to the hard view, HR strategies are about making corporate business strategies work – not overly adapting business strategies to take account of HR factors.

The soft approach focusses on the human side of HRM. People are a resource like any other, usually the most expensive, but they are the critical factor in turning other resources into valuable outputs. Creativity, commitment and skill can generate real competitive advantage. The *human* resource requires careful selection, nurturing and development, proper rewards and integration within the organisation. The availability or otherwise of relevant skills may cause business strategy to be altered. It assumes a unitary approach in terms of an organised team competing against other such teams. It tries to match the organisation's need for human resources with the individual's need for personal and career growth and development and to reduce costly turnover. The differences in the hard and soft approaches seem to be characterised more by questions of degree, based on values and beliefs about how people ought to be treated by organisations that need their skills, and what the real effect is on individual and collective performance in the longer term of different approaches to managing them, rather than an absolute opposites. Examples of Trusts operating at various points on this spectrum can be found but there is, to date, no evidence to demonstrate which type of approach leads to a better outcome.

Some years ago David Guest (1987) suggested that human resource management could be analysed in terms of four goals of integration, commitment, flexibility/adaptability and quality. Such adjectives are often used by senior NHS managers to describe the aims of their approach to HRM in their organisations but it is not always apparent that they all mean the same thing, or whether they would be pursued within a 'hard' or 'soft' approach.

Integration is achieved through viewing the workforce as a resource to be planned into the business development strategy. A distinction between this approach and the more traditional personnel management approach would be for the business to decide what it wants to do and only then turn around and look at the workforce and decide what might need to be done to gain employee commitment, how available skills might best be utilised or more likely, new skills developed, and what forms of agreement might have to be struck with the individual members of the workforce for the business to achieve its aims.

It is probably in terms of the goal of commitment that human resource management most greatly differs from that of traditional personnel management and underlines the unitary versus the pluralist perspective of human resource management. The policy objective here is for employees to have a much closer identity with the organisation in terms of its growth and prosperity. 'Committed employee behaviour rather than mere observance of formal procedure is, in many ways at the heart of human resource management'. (Storey 1989) HRM seeks to create an organisational state where individuals want to be associated with the organisation and to retain membership of it. In terms of the NHS this means individuals being identified with the achievement of specific objectives and targets as their contribution to the organisation's targets and objectives, and not to their profession or union or some other third party. HRM emphasises the development of individual contracts of employment in relation to the need for particular skills and most importantly in terms of reward for high performance.

The goal of flexibility and adaptability relates to the use of the workforce in a way that increases the ability of the organisation to respond quickly to any changes in its environment whether this be manifest in terms of the 'market', technological and scientific changes or other major interventions. This might be termed 'Darwinian management', where the ability to adapt quickly is the key to success and survival. Flexibility is demanded both in terms of the organisational structure and in terms of the workforce. Policy objectives would be aimed at reducing the influence of any third party body or organisation outside that which an individual works for, ie trades unions and professional organisations. Demarcation lines between professions and other skills and trades would need to be reduced if not removed.

The fourth goal of quality refers to the service or product and its delivery by the staff of the organisation, not only in terms of the need for the organisation as a whole to survive by delivering a quality service to its 'customer', but to build the image of the organisation in such a way that those currently belonging to it wish to remain because they identify with a recognised high quality employer. Recruitment opportunities are maximised because those outside the organisation will actively seek to join it because of its quality image, thus providing a better chance of getting the right people and matching people to jobs.

Of the many studies that have attempted to analyse and compare different approaches and identify core elements in HRM, three major elements emerge

1. the close integration of HRM and corporate strategy;

2. an employing organisation with a considerable degree of independence to take personnel decisions including an independent remuneration policy, allowing for a 'bottom line' focussed contingent pay policy and the absence of or at least minimal influence from trades unions;

3. preference for a carefully controlled, or in some conceptions, internal labour market; this would include freedom to recruit as the organisation

deems appropriate; absence or limitation of restrictions on employment contracts; and a substantial degree of training and development. (Brewer and Bournois 1991)

It was originally assumed that Trusts would have all of these freedoms. In reality there are situational constraints and there is no common model. It is increasingly obvious that Trusts must work out the detail of their own approach based on their own situational factors – which they must first be able to recognise. One unavoidable key element of human resource management is that it is not something left only to those with that job title. Given that human resource management, however defined, is a recognition from any organisation that its success is dependant upon its management of people, it is not something that can be left to specialists. It emphasises the line manager's need, whether working at the top strategic level of the organisation or at an operational/delivery level to manage their human resource in the most effective way they can. Kotter (1988) says that 'HR people have got to stop conceptualising their role as a "professional" individual contributor and realise that their job is to help provide corporations with leadership on HR issues . . . influencing other managers to take responsibility for finding, developing, retraining and motivating talent, and influencing them [line managers] to approach that responsibility in a sensible way'.

Performance management and human resource management

Managing the performance of Trusts whether at the level of the individual, group or team, directorate or whole organisation is critical to its success within the NHS. Nationally, increasing attention is being paid to this issue often in the belief that there is some panacea available based on a new technique or approach, as yet undiscovered. But it isn't quite like that. Taking a broad definition of performance management it probably encompasses that majority of processes and strategies that come under the definition of human resource management. Recent research on performance management (Bevan and Thompson 1992, Fletcher and Williams 1992) suggests that there is no consistent definition of performance management though organisations undertaking performance management are found to exhibit certain characteristics: They:

- have mission statements which are communicated to all employees;

- regularly communicate information on business plans and progress toward achieving these plans;

- implement policies such as total quality management (TQM) and performance related pay (PRP);

- focus on senior managers' performance rather than other manual and white collar employees;

- express performance targets in terms of measurable outputs, account-abilities and training/learning targets;

- use formal appraisal processes and CEO presentations as ways of communicating performance requirements;

- set performance requirements on a regular basis;

- link performance requirements to pay, particularly for senior managers.
  (Bevan and Thompson 1992)

Organisations vary widely in their use of the term performance management and Fletcher and Williams (1992) state that it is not used with a great deal of discrimination and that a number of the organisational representatives contacted in the course of their study simply did not know what performance management was, often perceiving it as another name for appraisal. There are a number of diagrammatic models around which describe a process of performance management, sometimes describing it as an ideal type. For example one model (Schneir 1989) puts individual performance appraisal at the centre of the performance management cycle and links individual goals and responsibilities to the objectives of the department or organisation, which is seen as the *start* of the process. The outcomes of the appraisal process are broken down into two broad human resourcing activities which affect the individual described as 'judging' and 'coaching'. Judging refers to issues such as compensation, succession planning and disciplinary measures, whereas coaching relates to means of improving performance through training and development and consideration of career options. But this is only one example.

Performance management is probably best thought of as a strategy which encompasses a wide range of factors relating to the management of performance in a particular organisation; basically, what performance outcomes are needed and what factors affect those outcomes.

First of all there must be an overall policy and strategy for the management of performance, second there must be a series of specific processes such as, but not only, individual appraisal which enable performance, third there needs to be a clear focus on the people in the organisation and finally the plant, equipment and physical environment in which they have to operate. All these factors are interdependent and must be approached in an integrated manner. They all contribute to the success or failure of the performance management system in an organisation. There are many examples of excellent individual processes such as well developed and sophisticated appraisal or reward strategies which still fail to achieve any real performance outcome because insufficient attention is paid to other factors in the equation. They are implemented and operated in isolation. In any organisation all factors must be geared to creating a shared vision of performance, generating commitment from employees to the concepts of improving performance and creating an environment where it is okay to perform. Shared vision is critical to the fulfilment of performance and this means that the vision and the concrete objectives that result from it must be communicated to all people in the organisation very clearly and in a manner which they can relate to their own particular role and tasks. It needs to generate some sense of purpose and commitment and give meaning. People need to understand how their efforts are of importance to the organisation.

Fundamentally, the performance management process in any organisation must be rooted in the business plan of that organisation. All factors must relate to the business goals and objectives and all performance outcomes from specific processes and activities associated with performance management must be measured against business criteria. Positive and involving feedback and communication on an individual, group or team and organisation-wide basis have to be continuous.

Many developments associated with performance management are reactions to specific stimuli within or outside the organisation which can often lead to a piecemeal and disintegrated approach with little clarity as to why particular processes or activities are being undertaken and how they might affect performance outcomes. The research referred to above suggests that organisations will experience greater success if they develop their policies with regard to all issues both internal and external rather than reacting to one particular pressure which can often create more problems than it solves. 'Performance management must be implemented strategically linked to commercial objectives with well thought through development phases and be focussed toward definite aims'. (IPM 1992)

One of the more contentious findings from some of the research was the doubt it cast upon the value of the pay-reward driven approach to performance management, ie performance related pay (PRP). This is particularly so where performance related pay policies were operated in a degree of isolation from other aspects of performance management. 'PRP, whilst a valuable tool in some respects, should be viewed realistically and not as the holy grail of increased performance'. (IPM 1992) It seems that the most appropriate role for PRP is as one of a number of components in a system of performance management and should be complementary rather than central to the performance management system.

Many systems designed to improve the effectiveness of the output and outcomes of health care organisations are too polarised around either a behavioural, organisation development approach or a rational data-led approach, in the way they are operationalised. The result is often ineffective in improving performance because it ignores one or other dimension. What is needed is a combining of both approaches, taking into account both the behavioural–organisation development approach to the management of individual and collective performance in organisations together with a hard data approach, which uses good quality management information to focus on key indicators of organisational performance, and is then able to link these back to both *what* is done by the people in the organisation and *how* they set about doing it. This combination of approaches into a single integrated approach is not common in the NHS or indeed in other organisations. Examples of NHS organisations with total quality management, resource management, medical audit, individual performance review, BS5750 etc can all be found to illustrate this point. These systems and processes are 'put into' organisations without a sufficiently clear sense either of their specific individual purposes or how they would integrate with other systems and processes within the organisation to produce a real performance outcome. Reductions achieved on waiting lists often revert once the immediate pressure is off because no self-sustaining system or new set of beliefs or procedures are put in place.

Many of these initiatives are developed in isolation from each other and where hard data is actually used, assuming it is available, and accurate etc, then different sets of data may well be developed for each of the different approaches, all measuring different aspects of performance with no coherent sense of common key indicators.

The various approaches are not integrated through the business plan or business strategy of the organisation in a way that ensures they support each other in the achievement of organisation or goals. If they were based on agreed and identifiable measures or organisational performance this would then enable an integrated and holistic approach to performance management utilising the different systems to achieve different aspects of performance but with all using the same core of performance measures. At the same time, if the effective assessment in measurement of performance is to lead to self generating performance improvements, then systems must motivate individual managers and staff in order to secure an improvement in individual departments and services. They must therefore encourage the development of appropriate beliefs and behaviours among managers and staff which sustain high performance for its own sake. Many NHS managers and professionals either do not have a performance orientation and or do not know how to use available information to measure individual or departmental/service performance.

As already discussed the developing literature on performance mangement systems underlines the development among those organisations that appear to be in the forefront of an integrated approach which not only combines different initiatives, but also focusses simultaneously on the interaction of individuals, groups or teams as well as the organisation as a whole, linked with both hard data and behavioural–organisation development approaches. The NHS is particularly bad at pigeon-holing separate approaches and initiatives, taking them as separate items on a very lengthy management agenda. It is innately geared to short-term thinking on performance issues. Health service organisations, particularly those at the provider level, need to explore and develop a holistic, strategic approach which combines a more effective tactical operation of the various systems currently available with securing a strategic improvement. It seems such a truism to say that an organisation's performance is dependent on the people in it. Yet the evidence available about what organisations actually do in practice when trying to implement systems and processes for performance improvement strongly imply that the opposite view prevails. Gaining a performance improvement is about getting individual people, whether working on their own or in groups or teams, to do things both better and differently in relation to what the organisation needs to remain competitive and successful. Individual systems and processes have to have meaning both in themselves and as part of a total approach. These ideas central to the concept of performance management, are at the heart of strategic human resource management.

The financial environment for the health service over the next few years will be particularly hostile and will further encourage fragmented short-term actions at national and local level to hold down costs while attempting to maintain outputs. Therefore if the NHS is to enter the 21st century in anything like reasonable shape there needs to be conscious opposition to fragmentation of effort and action and a very deliberate effort made to maintain a strategic focus on management of performance through effective management of human resources, ie the people of the NHS.

The changing roles and activities of human resource directors

Armstrong (1989), in a study of 20 personnel directors from large organisations, identified key issues in relation to the way the personnel department enables the management of human resources in an organisation:

1. The need to integrate the role of the personnel director and the human resource function into the business;

2. the emphasis on strategy;

3. the importance attached to treating the personnel function as an enabling one which is very much concerned with cultural and organisational change and with empowering people to improve their performance;

4. the increasing significance of resourcing activities at all levels of the organisation and that means resourcing in its broader sense – not only recruitment but also career management, development and performance related training;

5. the stress on performance, quality and customer care.

Armstrong's key issues describe the key characteristics of personnel/ human resource director posts at unit level. All responsibility for the operational organisation and delivery of health services has now been placed at unit level, with the appropriate organisation model being that of the NHS Trust. This is where the vast majority of the human resources of the NHS are located and so consequently will be the responsibility for their management. The role of regions though not yet finalised might still be one of broad strategic management on a co-ordinated regional–national basis. But this is by no means certain.

For the purchasers there may be a need for those at District level involved in the specifying and monitoring of contracts to assess the viability and quality of specifications being developed for services, and for bids against the specifications in terms of the human resource demands imposed by the contracts on any Unit seeking a contract. Will they be able to deliver? Have they got the right number of people with the right skills? Can they keep them? With a clear remit to ensure the long-term provision of high-quality services, effectively and efficiently delivered, purchasers may need to concern themselves in some detail with the long-term availability of people with the appropriate skills in the provider Units. This would require regular access to HRM advice and expertise of a high order, which could be contracted in from various sources, eg the increasing number of NHS based, independent consultants, academic-consultancy organisations or even other Units not in a provider relationship for health care services.

In the first and second wave Trusts' former District Directors often moved into the prospective Trust early on in the preparation, with Districts deliberately organising things so managerial time and resources could be released to concentrate on the preparatory work. (Though this is less obvious in third and fourth wave organisations, possibly because the pioneering work has now been done.) This underlined the refocussing of 'personnel or human resource activity' at unit level. The approach taken to the people issues of self-government generally reflects a strong 'human resource' management emphasis in contrast to the more traditional personnel emphasis. The trend appears to have been toward having higher quality, higher paid staff at Unit level but with a role based to a greater extent on enabling line managers to manage their own people better.

A survey of the key issues put forward by first wave Trusts revealed an emphasis on five areas, at that time:

1. the development and maintenance of a pay strategy;

2. training and developing all staff and managers for quality of service and higher performance;

3. human resource planning starting with the demand by Trusts for the skills they need to provide contracted services;

4. tackling the immediate and longer term recruitment, retention and return issues;

5. doctors' contracts and the range of 'new' medical staffing issues.

Comparing these issues with those put forward by Armstrong illustrates some significant differences of degree and emphasis but on the whole the overall role was described as more strategic in orientation with statements being made that everything must be geared to the business plan of the Trust. It was perhaps this attempt to take a more holistic approach to 'human resource' management as the way of enabling the new organisations to fulfil their more clearly understood and articulated core purpose, that distinguishes the new approach from the 'old' personnel management in the NHS. Though as many senior HR staff will admit, aspiration often exceeded reality.

At that time it was not certain whether the enthusiasm to adopt a 'leading edge' approach could be maintained and made more universal in the complexity of implementing the NHS reforms. What hadn't emerged at that time was a clear articulation of values which could provide a set of guiding principles for managing the people and make the difference between a set of new tricks that might, or might not, succeed and a basic philosophy of management that was to drive the new Trusts along and provide the measure against which they would judge and decide on the specific strategies to be adopted in managing the people of the trusts.

A more recent survey and general discussions with personnel and HR directors of Trusts around the current major issues and agenda items suggests the following in an approximate order of emphasis. They have been clustered around the ten key words used more frequently to describe the focus of various activities. The descriptions of the activities are based on phrases used by the directors. Most were described as integrating and overlapping with each other.

1. Culture
   — we are in the patient care business not the administration business
   — devolving internally, responsibility and accountability
   — decoupling from HAs, Regions and Whitley
   — defining purpose
   — clarity re 'the business'
   — more suited to a small business operation
   — greater personal accountability
   — greater sense of independence
   — no jobs for life

2. Flexibility
   — responding to purchasers
   — reduce demarcation
   — integration of the workforce
   — to develop and increase their (staff) effectiveness
   — remove career blockages
   — service led but people centred
   — increasing the application of the core and periphery (shamrock organisation) concept

3. Involvement — increasing the understanding and therefore the commitment of staff through developmental processes
    — looking for ways of involving consultants in management
    — increasing understanding of the nature of and need for change
    — involving trades unions in understanding the business
    — consultants (medical) managing projects
    — programmes to increase the loyalty to the organisation of professionals

4. Pay — increasing the use of job evaluation
    — going for a single pay spine
    — simplifying Whitley
    — relating it to business needs
    — national agreements less relevant
    — led by local financial concerns rather than central/political concerns

5. Productivity — have to control workforce costs
    — need to raise performance
    — manage sickness and absence to release £1m

6. Affordability — have to live on a contract income
    — managing the numbers of staff
    — looking at cheaper patterns of employment

7. Planning — planning the human resources need for the organisation
    — workforce profiling based on the numbers and skills needed to define services
    — planning how to downsize

8. Conflicts — consequence of major financial problems
    — dialogue with TUs
    — educating TUs about 'the business'
    — handling conflict caused by closures, redundancies and redeployment

9. Managers — line managers being accountable for managing their own staff
    — developing their own staff
    — need to develop line managers

10. Strategy — thinking longer term
    — a more strategic perspective

As can be seen there are clearly elements of HRM as described above, both hard and soft, but not all HR directors are fully involved in all the above. Local circumstances dictate the local agenda and the type of role undertaken. Much of Armstrong's work referred to at the beginning of this section is also reflected in the above. Comparison with the five areas identified by HR directors of first wave Trusts suggests that pay is possibly of lesser importance. This may reflect the early 'macho' approach displayed by some Trusts where pay was seen as a means of emphasizing independence and autonomy. Radicalism in pay for its own sake has no relevance unless it is part of a broader enabling process to create greater flexibility and productivity and performance in meeting contract requirements. Doctors' contracts seem to have dropped right out of sight as a specific issue. This is in some respects surprising given the central role of doctors on Trust performance. Proposals to change medical training and junior doctors' hours may put this back on the agenda.

On the whole any differences probably represent a greater and more measured understanding of the needs of provider organisations and in some cases a more sophisticated approach on the part of some HR directors based on the lessons of the last few years since the first wave Trusts came into being.

Effective management of the 'HRM' department

There are many broad national 'objectives', which coupled with a range of local issues provide a wealth of 'criteria' against which the effectiveness of the HR function might be judged, but they need to be turned into something much more specific and particular. Distinction should be made between the overall function in an organisation and the specialist department. The Personnel Standards Lead Body (1993) has set out a starting point for standards development against which the performance and effectiveness of a personnel department might be judged.

Effectiveness is unfortunately a subjective concept and depends on who defines it. People and organisations are effective if they meet the expectations of their bosses, subordinates, colleagues or customers. Sometimes, these expectations are set out in clear, agreed and precise objectives with clear performance standards and measures, but, more often, they are not. Either no attention is paid to objective setting or the process is not rigorous enough to ensure that the objective set for an organisation, the function or service, or an individual represents reality. The test is, will the pursuit and achievement of these objectives result in a consensus of opinion about the organisation, function, or person, as totally 'effective'? If the answer is no, then the objectives – the criteria for effectiveness – do not represent reality, as it is perceived by others.

Drucker defines effectiveness as 'doing the right things right', as against efficiency which is just 'doing things right'. Who decides what is right? Those providing the service or product, or those to whom it is provided? What are the assumptions and expectations of both parties? How explicit are they able to be in articulating them? Are they compared or tested?

Efficiency is frequently confused with effectiveness. A simplistic example for the human resource department might be that of an extremely fast and slick central recruitment administration system that puts people in jobs – square pegs in square holes – quickly. It is efficient at what it does. But, is there any clear sense of 'why' it is doing it, of what the organisational outcome will be? Should recruitment be aimed at obtaining octagonal or triangular pegs to enhance change? To recruit to fill vacancies quickly is fine, but what is the purpose of the recruitment process in terms of how it fits with other HR activities in meeting the business needs of the organisation? If there is no result in terms of any overall increase in organisational performance, however that might be defined in particular cases, then where does efficient recruitment take the organisation? Has anyone identified the skills needed to achieve a performance increase, or even what sort of performance increase is required and what it would mean in concrete measurable terms? Is there any link between what the organisation is trying to achieve and what human resources and skills it needs to do it? Should the HR department be doing it or should the line managers be handling their own recruitments? Only once it is clear 'why' recruitment is being undertaken, in terms of what contribution the recruitment process makes to the achievement of organisational goals and who should be doing it, can it be said we are 'doing the right thing'. Recruitment is a means to an end. This then provides measurable objectives and targets for the recruitment aspect of the human resource function in terms of both its efficiency and its effectiveness.

The same argument can be run for any other aspect of the human resource function such as training or employee relations or, indeed, for any other managerial function such as finance. Tyson and Fell (1986) define effectiveness for the personnel function in terms of 'the extent to which the members of the personnel department and the personnel policies give effect to the organisation's objectives', which presupposes clear organisational objectives. They suggest three areas in which judgements either are, or should be made:

1. the person;

2. the role and relationships of the function in the organisation;

3. contribution to strategic direction.

The first two are areas in which judgements are made every day both consciously and unconsciously by other individuals and departments and functions across the organisations. The third area is one in which judgements are usually not made, either because the organisation is one in which strategic focus and direction are hazy concepts to start with, or because the personnel specialist, or the rest of the organisation, or both, do not see the function in that light.

There are multiple expectations of any manager in an organisation and the personnel or human resource specialist is no exception. Often the effectiveness of the function is judged in terms of the perceived effectiveness of the most senior person in that function. Personal effectiveness is essentially a matter of being perceived as being effective in a particular job in a particular organisation at a particular time, ie an interaction of the person, the job and the organisation context. Such perceptions of effectiveness may be tied to measurable objectives, but equally may be impressionistic. Without clear, agreed and understood objectives, or a model of effectiveness, any perception of effectiveness will be based on whether or not an individual or indeed, their department of service, is meeting a rather vague set of 'expectations'. Within the interaction of the three variables, there are multiple factors influencing each of them, eg in terms of the person's experience, training, cognitive style and processes, competencies; in terms of the job demands, stated objectives, expectations, role and responsibilities; in terms of the organisation culture, nature of the business, environmental influences etc. The process leading to an outcome of 'effectiveness' on a personal level is complex. A manager needs the situational sensitivity to read and understand their particular situation. What are the expectations others have of me? Are they explicit or implicit? What do I have to do to be regarded as effective?

Having read the situation (hopefully accurately) then, in order to be considered effective, any manager must then be able to do something about meeting those expectations. The manager's behaviour has to be congruent with the expectations on him or her. The way the job is performed has to fit. If the manager, having identified what is expected of them decides that the expectations are inappropriate, either because they don't fit their own perception of what they should be doing, or what the organisation needs, or, they feel they haven't the ability to meet them, then they may want to renegotiate the expectations with others in the organisation. Again the way they go about this, their behaviour, must be congruent, ie acceptable. This assumes the manager has a range of skills of competencies that are organisation specific, ie they fit their particular organisational situation. Do HR specialists look to their own development with the same intensity that they might examine that of line managers?

Tyson and Fell (1986) bemoan 'the frequent absence of any rational judgement about the role of personnel' and that the 'problem of introducing new models of personnel is the problem of changing expectations'. As well as there being expectations held of any individual, there are more generalised expectations and assumptions, often untested, about what the human resource function is there for, or what its contribution could be. Sometimes, the 'vision' within the HRM function does not match the 'expectations' of the rest of the organisation. As with any individual manager, the effectiveness of any human resources function or department can be judged by its collective ability to bring into being a model of HRM which meets the needs of the organisation and, as a consequence, helps to structure the expectations of, and relationships with, the rest of the organisation that makes up its customers or clients.

John Humble (1988) suggests that HRM specialists should have a customer service orientation. Who are your customers? What do they want from you and what criteria do they use to judge you? Are their 'criteria' (expectations) different from your 'criteria' (assumptions)? How do you rate on their criteria?

The focus on identifying the expectations of others, and then setting out to either meet them or change them, does not mean abandoning any attempt to seek out objective measures of performance. But before they can be identified, there must be agreement about the nature and purpose of the function, leading to agreement on specific objective, and targets for measuring levels of performance and achieving those objectives. The assumptions and expectations of both the service providers and their customers must be tested and clarified. Knowing what perceptions the rest of the organisation has of you as a function, and as individuals, is important, because that image or perception will govern behaviour and attitude toward the HRM function. Asking your customers to provide the criteria, by which your service should be judged, could be quite salutary. Comparing your rating of your service or department on their criteria with their rating could be even more salutary!

The HRM function should set out to market itself not sell itself. Marketing is to do with meeting the needs of the customer. Selling is to do with meeting the needs of the seller. This might mean that some of the aspirations of the human resource function and the people in it may have to be held in check. This does rely on the capability of any given human resource department and the people in it to deliver, it does not mean that the vision has to be trimmed or reduced or that it should be abandoned as a hopeless ideal. There is a balance to be achieved between world domination and stagnation!

Contributing to strategic direction and policy represents a higher level of judgement about any managerial function. By definition, it must be based on a deliberate and conscious strategic process, rather than on impressionistic judgements. At the beginning of this chapter the foundations of success for any organisation were discussed, ie a clear mission or vision constantly reviewed, clearly articulated, and based on a set of high performance people-centred values, governing everything the organisation does in pursuit of its vision. If these fundamentals are lacking in an organisation, then it will be difficult for any objective judgement to be made about the effectiveness of the HRM function, or, indeed, any other function, in terms of its contribution to strategy. HRM specialists may set out to influence their organisation to take this route to success to be more strategic and, in doing so, not only establish their role but ensure their strategic contribution.

Some of the difficulties and issues facing the NHS up to the end of the century and beyond have been touched on in this chapter and elsewhere in the book. Public sector organisations have some particular difficulties in setting clear strategic objectives and in maintaining a sustained effort and focus on them, which makes it difficult for any individual manager or managerial function to keep a long-term vision in focus. HRM specialists must be in the business of trying to facilitate organisational clarity in terms of purpose and direction, and ensuring HRM policies and procedures are coherent and supportive in their pursuit – subject to the provisos about capacity, capability and pace referred to above.

The HRM department may have to reconcile its own aspirations with what its customers want and to reconcile both with what the organisation needs. This assumes that it has the capability to assess organisational need. If the HRM department has no concept of its potential role in the fundamental success of the organisation, then it can never be effective, it may be efficient. The key purpose of personnel is to 'enable management to enhance the individual and collective contributions of people to the short and long term success of the enterprise'. (Personnel Lead Body 1993)

Chief executives interviewed by the Lead Body criticised personnel directors who were over concerned with rules and procedures, introduced systems and procedures which didn't fit business needs and took an indiscriminate approach to being a good employee. To be effective senior personnel professionals needed to gain respect by demonstrating a real contribution to the business, be able to 'read the organisation' for the chief executive, assist in developing individual and team performance and exercise judgement in supporting and opposing executive actions. The personnel department must be seen to be businesslike and ready to meet the same pressures as the rest of the organisation. Its own management must be an exemplar and identify the critical factors against which its own success can be measured.

The study by David Guest of the effectiveness of personnel in the NHS concluded that effectiveness was highest in those units where there is a close partnership between personnel and line management involving

1. a clear articulation and integration of personnel policies and goals of the top level of the organisation;

2. a high level of joint senior management team influence over major organisational decisions;

3. a high level of process effectiveness among personnel staff.
   (Guest and Peccei 1992)

Size and type of unit or the size and resources of the personnel department were not directly linked to effectiveness and neither was the degree of professionalisation. Primarily it was the development of a closer partnership with line managers and all that implies in terms of the personnel department's approach that decided whether or not the department was perceived as effective.

The potential contribution the HRM function, led by HR specialists, can make to the successful delivery of health care is vast because it is about people providing services to other people. Those in the specialist department must develop the situational sensitivity to recognise where the opportunities are and where the short-term limitations of 'the systems' or the capacity or capability of the organisation, or indeed the department itself, require the exercise of patient persistence in working toward the long-term vision.

In the final analysis, the effectiveness of the specialist HRM department can be judged in terms of the extent to which line managers are empowered and enabled to manage their own human resources and the extent to which they are successful at it. HRM specialists should take the view that managing the people of the organisation is too important to be left to them. It must be something that all line managers want to do, and to do as well as possible. The role of the HRM specialist is to provide the leadership and the inspiration that encourages line managers to want to do it well. If 'personnel' or 'HRM' is seen as 'something that the personnel department does', then managing the people who are the health service's human resource will not be given the prominence needed for the NHS to survive as a successful organisation in the 1990s. The people with the scarce skills we need will go elsewhere unless the NHS with its million plus staff tries, as far as it can, to be a trend-setter in terms of valuing people and providing them with a dignified working environment that recognises their desire for a better quality of life, and a synergy between home and working life. In doing so the purpose of the health care organisation must never be forgotten so that there is equally a synergy between organisational need and individual needs. The needs of the organisation, ie the business of providing health services to people, should predominate but, decisions affecting the life and livelihood of individuals must be taken in line with a set of values which are well known and credible to all in the organisation. These should enable even the redundant employee to feel that even in such unpleasant circumstances they have been treated with dignity and with a reasonable concern for their material well-being. Is this too sophisticated a challenge for the human resource specialists to throw down before the line managers?

References

Armstrong M 1989 'Personnel directors view from the bridge' *Personnel Management* Oct, Institute of Personnel Management

Bevan and Thompson 1992 *An overview of Policy and Practice in performance management in the UK* Institute of Personnel Management

Brewster and Bournois 1992 'Human Resource Management: A European Perspective' *Personnel Review* 20 (6) MCB

Buller PF 1988 'Successful partnerships: HR and strategic planning of eight top firms' *Organisational dynamics* Autumn

Clutterbuck D and Crainer S 1988 *The Decline and Rise of British Industry* W H Allen and Co

Donovan 1968 *Royal Commission on Trade Unions and Employers Associations Report* Cmnd 3623 HMSO, London

Drucker P 1990 *Managing the Non-Profit Organisation* Butterworth-Heineman

Fletcher and Williams 1992 'Organisational Experience' *Performance Management in the UK* Institute of Personnel Management

Fredman S and Maurice G 1989 'The state as employer: setting a new example' *Personnel Management* Aug, Institute of Personnel Management

Garratt 1987 *The Learning Organisation* Fontana

Goldsmith W and Clutterbuck D 1984 *The Winning Streak* Weidenfeld and Nicholson, London

Gowler and Legge 1986 'Images of employees in company reports – do company chairmen view their most valuable asset as valuable?' *Personnel Review* **15**, 5

Guest D 1987 'Human resource management and industrial relations' *Journal of Management Studies* **24**, 5

Guest D and Peccei R 1992 'Measuring Effectiveness: in NHS Personnel Getting it Right *Health Manpower Management* **18** (4) MCB

Harvey-Jones J 1988 *Making it Happen* Collins, Glasgow

Harvey-Jones J 1992 *Trouble Shooter* Collins, Glasgow

Humbe J 1988 'How to Improve the Personnel Service' *Personnel Management* Feb Vol 20, Institute of Personnel Management

Institute of Personnel Management 1992 *Conclusions in Performance Management in the UK* Institute of Personnel Management

Kanter RM 1984 *The Change Masters* Allen and Unwin, London

Klein R 1982 'Performance, evaluation and the NHS: A case study in conceptual perplexity and organisational complexity' *Public Administration* **60**, 385–40. Royal Institute of Public Administration, London

Kotter J 1988 *The Leadership Factor* Macmillan

Management and Personnel Office 1987 *Working Patterns* a study document by the Cabinet Office

National Health Service Training Authority 1985 *Better Management, Better Health*

Personnel Standards Lead Body 1993 *A Perspective on Personnel* Department of Employment

Peters T and Watermann R 1982 *In Search of Excellence* Harper and Row

Schneir CE 1989 'Implementing Performance Management and Recognition and Rewards at the Strategic Level: A Line Management Driven Effort' *Human Resource Planning* **12** (3)

Senge P 1990 *The Fifth Discipline: The Art and Practice of the Learning Organisation* Century, London

Stewart and Ranson 1988 'Management in the public domain' *Public Money and Management* **8**(1) and **8**(2). Basil Blackwell, Oxford and New York

Storey S 1989 'Human resource management in the public sector' *Public Money and Management* Autumn. Basil Blackwell, Oxford and New York

Torrington D 1988 'How does human resource management change the personnel function?' *Personnel Review* **17**

Tyson S and Fell A 1986 *Evaluating the Personnel Function* Hutchinson

8 Buying and selling high-quality health care

Hugh Koch

The essence of excellence is the thousand concrete, minute actions performed by everyone in an organisation to keep a company on course.

Tom Peters

Introduction

Searching for quality in health care and the defining of the process of assuring and managing quality has a certain timelessness to it. Florence Nightingale was perhaps one of the first modern managers (written about so often in recent American management texts) who 'managed by walking about' (MBWA). She, no doubt, had a complex set of standards in her mind, some unconscious, some intuitive and some very obvious as she walked her wards. Then, as now, the issue of how such standards have their own qualities of being 'explicit, operational, measurable, and consumer-centred' was, and is, crucial. This chapter will, in part, address how health care standards can be set within a total corporate context in which all staff feel ownership for quality management. In addition, the implementation of the *Working for Patients* legislation has had, as one of its main planks, the introduction of market forces and the contracting process to 'push up' quality of health care, and the implications and mechanisms of this will be outlined.

Quality health care in context

Over a relatively short period of time, many public and private sector companies and services have focussed upon quality as an essential ingredient for successful development and survival. They have endeavoured to incorporate quality processes into every aspect of their operations. To do this has meant fundamental changes in the way

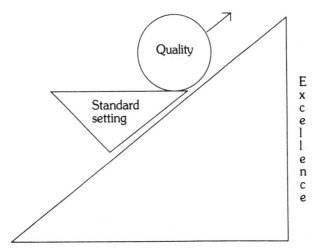

Figure 8.1 Quality ball 'on the hill'

managers and staff perceive their work. Quality became a top strategic issue in the 1980s in Europe, Japan and the USA.

Health care quality in the 1970s and early 1980s was maintained and guarded predominantly by the health care professionals themselves, highly trained people who practised their many and varied skills 'to the standards they had been taught' – to question their consistency in doing so was often not thought appropriate. This, coupled with occasional external investigative bodies, eg HAS, ENB, ensured that, on the positive side, many hospitals were operating high-quality services to patients, and, on the negative side, quality was inconsistent, patchy and poorly defined, and randomly improved upon.

With the Introduction of the Griffiths Recommendations for General Management (1983), the issue of quality assurance was placed firmly and uncompromisingly on the general manager's agenda, ensuring he/she was tasked through the IPR appraisal process to define, monitor and review standards of care and service throughout a District, Unit or hospital. The process, illustrated in Figure 8.1 of assessing current standards, ensuring their maintenance and improvement, had started.

With the implementation of *Working for Patients* recommendations, quality of care has become a focal point, at times controversially so, among 'providers' (hospitals, Trusts, clinicians), 'purchasers' (Commissioning Agencies, FPCs) and patients (general public). The traditional reliance on the professions to measure quality has rapidly been complemented by a business-style environment characterised by purchasers' ability to obtain value for money, providers' ability to differentiate themselves on the basis of quality of health care, and the general public's capacity to understand, and select, optimal and effective health care treatment alternatives.

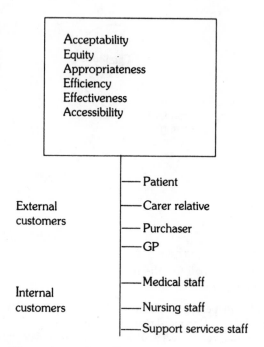

Figure 8.2   Dimensions of quality

Definition of quality

Difficult to define, but by no means impossible. Figure 8.2 illustrates
several parameters by which quality can be defined (and subsequently
measured).

This model partly rests on Robert Maxwell's (Director of the King's
Fund) six dimensions of quality: *acceptability, equity, appropriateness,
efficiency, effectiveness and accessibility.* Of all these, the first is
undoubtedly the 'driving force' of the others, or very rapidly will
become so. The ability to provide any service which meets the patients'
needs or expectations or is seen to make stupendous efforts towards
this will be a major quality predictor of success. These dimensions
apply in turn to the *care/service* itself, *information* given or elicited,
the way this is *communicated*, and the *attitude* of the communicator,
and the physical *environment* in which this is achieved. Again, of all
these, a major predictor of success will be the consumer orientation to
eliciting information to encourage and bring about customer/patient
responsibility in the care process. The responsibility for the above
does not rest with one individual, or even with a collection of

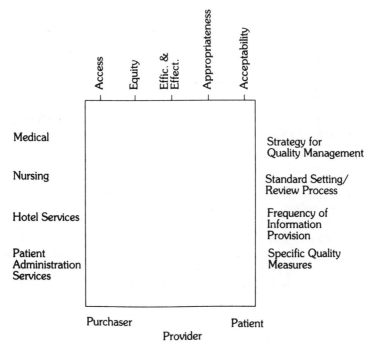

Figure 8.3   Quality specification categories

individuals, it rests with *every individual* member of staff, irrespective of the extent of their direct patient contact, each *department* or *specialty*, each *multidisciplinary team*, all levels of *management*, and rests fundamentally with the overall *culture* which the hospital develops.

Clearly, the predominant aim of any service is to its 'external' customer, the patient, his/her relatives, GP and purchasing agency. A second aim is to ensure a quality environment and culture for the service's staff – its 'internal' customer.

Specification of quality for purchasers, providers and patients

Setting aside the problematic issue of measuring whatever quality parameters are chosen, there is still confusion about which parameters are the most relevant to consider and monitor. The consumers need to be able to measure the quality of hospital A versus hospital B for a particular procedure or service. This partly rests on gaining access to, and making use of, information which is already available (eg waiting times, cross-infection rates, length of stay). It also rests on helping the recipient of such information to understand it and understanding its implication (Peat Marwick Main 1988). The information required for quality of service will differ depending on the recipient (eg purchaser, provider manager, or patient), but will largely fall into categories illustrated in Figure 8.3.

The provider will increasingly be expected by a purchaser to:

1. have a comprehensive strategy for providing quality services within a total quality management framework;

2. have a systematic approach and plan for establishing, monitoring and reviewing standards of care and service;

3. be able to provide information by specialty or service on pertinent quality variables on a regular basis.

Most providers will find little or less difficulty in furnishing purchasers with 'process' information on quality, eg the level to which consumers are central to care. However, the whole area of 'health outcomes' is one which, at present, creates great difficulty for the provider. However, as medical and nursing audit with or without technological support (eg Medical Data Index MDI or Ward FIP) develops, information should become more readily available (Shaw 1992).

Standard setting of health care quality

There are very few well-defined sets of standards in health care available for purchasers, providers or patients. There has been, relative to other industries, a relative reluctance by staff and managers to state such standards explicitly. Traditionally, providers of health care have, using the examples of doctors and nurses, viewed quality as two-dimensional: technical care and quality of 'expressive care'. Technical care includes diagnostic and therapeutic elements, expressive care includes provision of information and style of communication.

Purchasers, providers and patients have differing expectations about how to define, measure, and control quality. Balancing these expectations and developing an approach that encompasses each viewpoint is essential. Whatever method of definition of service/care standards is used, the most practical way to balance these expectations is to ensure patients and the general public have better information about quality of service provided. Quality information for the public will have several purposes:

1. It will provide more objective criteria for defining and measuring quality.

2. It will facilitate the comparison of providers on the basis of quality.

3. It will assist the patient/public/consumer to make informed choices about treatment alternatives.

4. It will stimulate health care professionals to improve the quality of care.

Where are hospitals now in terms of standards setting? Anyone walking the corridors of a hospital and enquiring of staff or even departmental heads how their quality of service is defined, maintained and improved will, at the present time, not find many cogent replies. This 'acid test' of staff's involvement in the quality process will change. However, what has occurred in many hospitals is the attempt to define standards using typically the structure–process–outcome model. *Structure* includes the resources inputted to a service (eg numbers of staff, level of training, availability of policies and procedures). *Process* includes the way in which the service is provided (eg staff training, information and communication processes, adherence to policies and procedures). *Outcome*, the most important and relevant of the three variables, includes items by which the service could be evaluated by the consumer (eg level of cross-infection, promptness and appropriateness of care, accidents to patients or staff, outcome of operation).

The process of defining structure/process/outcome characteristics has several important elements to it.

1. It has to be developed as much as is possible by the staff it will apply to. Many feel that staff have to have a crucial involvement in defining standards if they are to be committed to maintaining them. A slow, gradual process.

2. The definition of outcomes is considerably more difficult than defining the structure and process of care. To define outcome numerically and behaviourally is fraught with difficulty at present.

3. The definition process is repeatable, at least annually, as the process immediately releases new insights into the standard of care in greater depth.

4. The process should be applied to all services irrespective of size, closeness to patient, or relative status, and all elements of care (ie inpatient, daypatient, outpatient, domiciliary) should be addressed.

Standard setting, within a total quality management framework, has been attempted in several hospitals covering both priority services (eg Somerset Mental Health Services) and acute services (eg Dudley Acute Services). The several dimensions are summarised in Figure 8.4.

As indicated in the central part of the diagram, quality management via standard setting involves monitoring performance of services against set standards, setting improvement targets and establishing a regular annual review of performance.

The standard setting discussed above is primarily provider-centred. Two other sources of standard setting have emerged, these relate to purchaser-centred standards and options for accreditation by external source (not specifically related to *Working for Patients* recommendations).

Purchaser-centred standard setting emanates increasingly from local

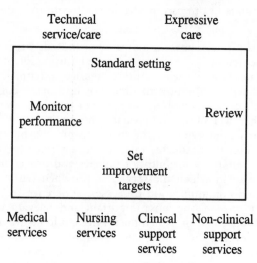

Figure 8.4   Standard setting framework

networking undertaken by the purchasing agency in order that it can be 'assured' of the quality of service provided by units with which it has placed contracts. The agency networks with a variety of consumers – patients, relatives, general practitioners, other statutory and voluntary agencies interfacing with the providers to elicit 'consumer feedback' as to the quality of services being purchased.

External accreditation is a mechanism for establishing what organisational standards, systems and processes relating to the delivery of healthy care are in place in any particular Unit/Hospital. The evaluation of compliance with explicit standards is by means of a survey carried out by a team of health care professionals, and has the advantage of being independent and able to use national standards as important reference points. The King's Fund have been leading the way in the UK in accreditation (King's Fund 1988). In the South Western Region, a 'small hospitals' accreditation board has already been established (NAHA 1988).

Quality strategy for provider Units

Each provider Unit should clearly state its aims and objectives for ensuring quality of service provided to one or more purchaser:

1. It should have a coherent programme for the systematic development and monitoring of quality improvement and management across all disciplines.

2. It should seek to develop an increased quality awareness *culture* amongst staff in all areas.

	1991/92	Predicted 1992/93	Quarter I Pred. Act. Var.	Quarter II Pred. Act. Var.	Quarter III Pred. Act. Var.	Quarter IV Pred. Act. Var.	Cumulative Pred. Act. Var.
Activity (Bed days) Hospital A Hospital B Total							
Expenditure (£000) Nurse staffing Drugs MSE							
Quality Waiting time LOS Readmission rate Complaints							

Figure 8.5   Workload agreement: general surgery

3. It should ensure the development of a coherent set of quality standards covering process and outcome of service across *all* specialties and departments, using quality assessment tools which are comprehensive, quantitative and capable of being used comparatively between location/hospitals over time.

4. It should ensure the management process is in place to monitor and develop the achievement of quality standards set, and hence improvements.

5. It should ensure information *provided* to patients is of high quality.

6. It should ensure effective mechanisms are in place to elicit, and act upon, information obtained from patients via complaints, surveys, suggestion schemes, user-groups.

7. It should ensure accurate specification of quality variables in management contracts with purchaser(s).

8. It should ensure accurate specification of quality variables in clinical contracts/workload agreements between Unit/Trust management and consultants.

In respect of workload agreements, Figure 8.5 illustrates the type of information, specifically quality, which is, in many hospitals, currently being developed.

At present, such quality information is fairly crude. However, this will rapidly develop and will also be further subdivided into Clinically Related Categories (CRCS).

Total quality management

Staff and managers in the NHS have always tried to improve the quality of service in their own way – new ideas and techniques come and go: quality becomes inconsistent in some areas: enthusiasm wanes – so what can really ensure quality management transcends the vagaries and changes in hospitals? Recently, the concept, strategy and action of *total quality management* has been introduced to the NHS and is destined to have dramatic effects on health care delivery in the UK (Touche Ross 1990). During 1989/90, the Department of Health made funds available for 17 TQM Demonstration sites to begin to develop TQM strategy and action plans. But what is it?

Total quality management is an approach which enables a hospital/ Unit/Trust to improve its ability to meet patient/customer requirements through a coordinated programme of quality review and improvement involving all staff, at whatever grade or seniority. Key elements of the approach are:

- developing a spirit or culture of continuous improvement and willingness by all staff to accept positive, healthy changes;

- identifying ways of establishing what patient/consumers want and improving hospitals' ability to respond to these;

- establishing, maintaining and reviewing key quality standards;

- establishing multi-disciplinary action teams to improve quality;

- eliciting staff's inbuilt motivation and inherent good sense to improve the service;
- strong managerial and clinical leadership.

It rests on the fundamental belief that focussed and corporate management action can lead to improved quality of care and service. This, in turn, leads to distinctive quality at competitive cost and hence satisfied customers and growth in health care market share (PA Consulting Group 1989).

TQM must be:

- *Management led* – Top management cannot expect staff to take quality responsibilities seriously if it does not do so itself. Senior managers and clinicians must give a clear lead to their staff on quality issues.

- *Unit/hospital wide* – Piecemeal improvements can be as counterproductive as they are useful. Enduring improvement in quality comes from all staff in all departments playing equal parts.

- *Everyone's responsibility* – Managers, departmental heads and consultants need to convince all their subordinates that quality is critical to the hospital's viable future and to the security of their jobs.

- *Prevention not detection philosophy* – despite frequently spending more on prevention, this is usually compensated adequately for by a fall in overall 'quality costs'.

- *'Right first time' standard* – Delegation for quality to the staff providing the care and service results in concentration on doing the job well and getting it right first time.

- *Cost of quality control* – Apart from opportunity costs, ie health care markets lost due to poor quality (becoming more identifiable through cross-boundary flow), the internal cost of quality can be assessed more easily now. The 'failure' costs (eg equipment breakdown, sickness/absence etc) can be calculated relatively easily. The cost of the service we develop to protect the patient/customer from these, the 'appraisal' costs (eg agency staff, management time) can also be assessed. Added to this are the 'prevention' costs.

- *Continuous improvement* – Meeting patients' needs and requirements is an evolutionary and continuous process. Our 'best' today is inevitably 'not quite enough' tomorrow. Staff should seek out improvements and accept ownership of quality problems as they arise.

Process of total quality management

The four main phases in introducing and sustaining TQM in a hospital/Unit/Trust are:

1. Assessment of current situation – this aims to 'diagnose' a Unit's present performance in terms of quality and agree a quality improvement programme for the unit. It involves:

   - ascertaining consumer views on services provided;
   - increasing awareness by staff of need for improvements;
   - building commitment at all levels to improve quality;
   - creating a new understanding of the need for inter-departmental teamwork;
   - establishing need to set standards for measuring and improving performance;
   - selected in-depth studies of one or two specific problems.

2. Management commitment – TQM means a significant shift in management style and practice. This shift can only take place if senior management takes the lead. Workshops for senior managers help to think through and plan how to coordinate and control quality improvement, and how each manager will involve his own department in the improvement process. At the end of this phase, every senior manager should own, and be accountable for, the TQM process for his department. Managerial leadership, performance and behaviour will be under the microscope by their staff.

3. Planned quality improvement – This aims to build awareness and commitment throughout the hospital and put in place practical mechanisms for achieving improvement. These include:

- quality action teams (eg reduce waiting times for outpatients; improve visitor facilities);
- standard setting;
- departmental action programmes (ie current form/shortcomings/ action plan/implement);
- systems design;
- staff development.

This process involves a major communications programme to make all staff aware of the TQM programme and obtain their commitment to it, and includes inter-disciplinary workshops for departmental heads and team briefings. This aims to give and elicit information.

To direct and monitor TQM programme and ensure continuous, sustained improvement, a support structure is needed comprising:

- a total quality steering group including the UGM/chief executive, other UMB officers and chairman of medical executive committee or staff committee;
- a total quality officer/coordinator to manage the ongoing process.

4. Positive feedback – To ensure the focus on quality does not become a 'flavour of the month' which passes, it is essential to:

- quantify successes and identify next steps;
- validate internal perceptions of success via customer feedback;
- ensure all staff get feedback, whether or not involved;
- involve more staff in setting new quality goals;
- encourage integration of management quality objective setting with staff enthusiasm and commitment.

Total quality management in the 1990s

Hospitals and Trusts will need to place a high emphasis on quality as a central element of their business plan. This should not, and cannot, just be a passing fancy but must instead involve a fundamental re-shaping of their corporate priorities for providing health care worth purchasing. The reasons for this attitude are:

1 The likely success of hospitals taking quality seriously

With the availability of choice of services to a purchaser, especially a large aggregation of old-style DHAs and FPCs, hospitals/Trusts offering services, which are not only cost-efficient but provide explicit quality, will attract contracts for cross-boundary care away from hospitals whose emphasis on quality is less. In five to ten years from now, the differential quality of care which already exists will be reflected in financial viability and capital development/reduction.

2 Rising expectations of customers

The public – the patient, their relative or carer – are becoming increasingly more informed as to how the quality of care can be defined and how it can vary. What might have been acceptable a decade ago, is becoming less acceptable now and, in the brave new world of contracting, the public will expect the health care purchased on their behalf to be of higher standards yet. Hospital services will expand not only because of the actual service standard but also because patient/customer expectations, having been raised, are being fulfilled and met.

3 The concentration by purchasers on quality-conscious providers

Purchasers will realise that to focus attention on *working with* providers to improve quality will pay off. The trend will be to contract with one or two main providers, not necessarily the local provider, for a longer period of time, and to expect more of them. Purchasers will not only look at the contract price, but will obviously consider quality, access and effectiveness and the overall quality management system which providers have developed. Providers faced with this situation will have little choice but to focus totally on quality – this will for the 'successful' provider lead to sustained growth in the available health care market.

4 Cost advantage of providing quality

Quality problems in health care provision are expensive. Waste of time and resources 'putting things right' can account for a significant proportion of revenue in any typical hospital. At present, these costs are rarely systematically identified – once clarified, however, these released resources can be re-invested in further quality improvements.

The advantages/benefits of introducing quality management are many and varied, and include:

1. Improved hospital image – lower complaint rates, higher satisfaction.

2. Improved throughput – elimination of service 'blockages' ensuring smoother and more rapid patient flows.

3. Cost/price reductions – savings in operational costs through greater focus on quality.

4. Improved morale   – staff in quality hospital, with a reputation
                            for this quality, will want to stay and
                            will enjoy doing so.

5. Improved management   – by adopting explicit standards,
                            managers will make better decisions
                            more frequently.

6. Committed purchasers   – Quality service provided to the customer
                            (via the purchaser) will result in both
                            customer and purchaser creating a part-
                            nership with the hospital based on
                            mutual trust.

Conclusions

One of the most crucial elements of the *Working for Patients* legislation
is the distancing of the purchaser of health care from those providing it.
The positive influence that a purchaser can bring to bear on a provider,
not least in terms of ensuring he can 'buy' high-quality health care and
service, will be of inestimable value – the extent to which this 'positive
influence' is accompanied by a real threat of contracts *not* being placed
where they currently would be expected will determine, probably, the
change in quality achieved. The market force can at long last be, in some
cases, truly felt and truly effective in the consumer's – the patient's,
your and my – best interest.

As important as the purchaser/provider issue, the move of managers
towards a total quality management, philosophy and approach, which
was occurring in any case, irrespective of the new legislation, is a very
positive move towards service improvement, and will bring the NHS in
line with other successful companies who have, since 1950, assimilated
a total quality philosophy into their operations.

References

Cheltenham and District Health Authority (1990) *Total Quality
    Management in Acute Services* Cheltenham.
Kings Fund Centre (1988) *Health Services Accreditation* London.
Koch, HCH (1991) *Total Quality Management in Health Care*
    Longman.
Koch, HCH (1991) *Exceeding Expectations. TQM in Mental Health
    Services Training Pack* Pavilion Publishing, Brighton.
Koch, HCH (1992) *Implementing and Sustaining TQM* Longman.
NAHA (1988) *Towards Good Practices in Small Hospitals* London.
PA Consulting (1989) *How to Take Part in the Quality Revolution*
    Bowater House, London.
Peat Marwick Main & Co. (1988) *Setting Quality Standards in Health
    Care* London.

Shaw, CD (1992) *Specialty Medical Audit* Kings Fund.
Somerset Health Authority (1988) *Quality Assurance of Mental Health Services* Taunton, Somerset.
Touche Ross (1990) *Personal Communication* London.

9 Implications of the NHS reforms for the future of primary health care in the United Kingdom

David Schofield and Peter Hatcher

Introduction

At a time when primary health care (PHC), as a concept and in practice, is identified as being at the very heart of health care and health service development, both internationally, and in the UK, there is commensurate emphasis being attached to the need for enhancing the capabilities of those individuals and groups with the responsibility for efficient and effective management of PHC. Research findings and reported experience of international organisations concerned with health and social development working closely with governments and communities (Ebrahim and Ranken 1988) strengthen such arguments – consistently and patiently stated and restated by such as the World Health Organisation (WHO 1989b) – and, in the UK, these emphases have been brought to the fore by way of government initiatives to prioritise the improvement of PHC services through their White Papers and consultation documents: *Promoting Better Health*, and *Working for Patients, Health of the Nation* and *Caring for People*. These are now being implemented under the National Health Service and Community Care Act 1990.

The discussion here attempts to assess the potential of these NHS reforms for effective PHC and the implications for their management, particularly through the new Family Health Service Authorities (FHSAs), formerly FPCs, in relation to the consistent guidelines for PHC as set down, as modified through experience, and practised with some success in other international contexts.

It is not uncommon for the concepts behind comprehensive PHC to be viewed as rather idealistic and impractical. This view is coincidentally rather convenient for governments since it enables them to continue determining (and controlling) health policy at a centralist level. Experience overseas of PHC programmes suggests there are two critical features: 1 a community orientation and 2 inter-sectoral collaboration.

The first of these is crucial, and sees local communities defining, planning and controlling services to meet their own health needs. In order to create such an approach, a number of factors need to alter. Governments must be willing to relinquish centralised control, and to allow local communities to define their own requirements. There also needs to be a shift of emphasis away from secondary, specialist, high cost care focussed upon rectifying illness towards a more integrated preventive strategy. Professional staff need to change traditional views, become more flexible in patterns of service delivery (including enhanced inter-sectorial collaboration) and to acknowledge a valid input from the community in decisions about health care priorities.

A critical question in the UK is how far the newly constituted management of FHSAs has provided the direction and leadership to develop a comprehensive PHC system? How far has government policy facilitated such development? The remainder of the chapter will focus upon how FHSAs have so far interpreted their new role and especially how they have implemented the White Paper requirements, and the implications for the future of PHC within a UK national health system. A key aspect is the degree to which change has been engendered in the attitude of professional staff; the following are examples of the issues that need to be tackled.

1. The effect of the rigid professionalism in formal health services needs to be minimised in order to maximise the flexibility essential to allow the development of community-oriented skills in health workers.

2. Nurture in professional health staff a new tradition of allowing communities to become involved with them in the decision-making process.

3. Nurture in professional health staff a new assumption that knowledge possessed by the community regarding their own health situation may not be compatible with modern medical/scientific traditions and yet is wholly appropriate as informal knowledge towards enhancing the health of the community.

4. Nurture in formal professional health organisation and in non-professional health staff a new flexibility, and willingness, to think about things, analyse things and do things in different, less 'traditional' and yet more effective ways.

This re-orienting of health practice, by dis-enfranchising health service staff from traditional entrenched professional values and beliefs, to develop methods for ensuring community participation in health activities, constitutes the real challenge for those managers committed to a comprehensive health care system for all, and, from the outset, requires opportunities to be created whereby the community and health service staff workers establish a basis for future partnership.

FHSAs and information for PHC

The White Paper *Working for Patients* offers a real opportunity for FHSAs to:

- identify community health issues, problems and needs as the essential basis for broad, integrated, district-based PHC programme planning, implementation and evaluation;

- identify those areas within their auspices which suffer from under-provision of general medical, dental and pharmacy services, for purposes of re-allocation of human/professional resource to suit real community health needs;

- review, prioritise and update PHC programme elements in terms of their appropriateness to local needs;

- identify which elements are specifically, and realistically, within the brief of FHSAs, breaking them down into more detailed FHSA service sub-elements, and incorporating into that process an assessment of different sectors responsibility for, or involvement in, the different elements. This has particular relevance for FHSAs in their interaction with, and in their role as, motivators of interaction between such sectors, for example, as local representative committees of the contractor professionals, CHCs, DHAs, local authorities etc.

Quite rightly, *Working for Patients* emphasises the value of more sophisticated FHSA patient registers as being a valuable information base for DHAs to, more effectively, identify and contact target populations for screening and surveillance programme development and, generally, for more effective health service planning. However, the real opportunity presented here to FHSAs would be one of coordinating information as a support to the whole management process essential for the broader concept of primary health care, as detailed above, to work in practice. Patient registers offer some evidence of health trends as presented in GPs' and dentists' surgeries and can form the basis of more selective health care provision. More relevant would be a wide range of information whereby a District level health profile would be developed, highlighting health status issues and 'patch' health needs by means of epidemiological, demographic etc, data. This would form the basis of an essential review of current activity, highlighting quality and quantity of health service provision, lack of provision and/or inappropriateness of provision. The development of a district level profile of relevant and appropriate sector support would serve FHSAs both to help develop the health profile, review current activity and also help develop policy for the realignment of activity to suit community health needs. Both White Papers emphasise how FHSAs are in a position to take responsibility for the development of an information system for PHC strategy development and implementation, especially in their role as 'networkers' across FHSs, DHAs and RHAs. A comprehensive FHSA database, used for patient registration, screening, service planning etc, would form the basis of an FHS/NHS network. The success of a comprehensive primary health care system relies on a National Health Service-wide strategy to enable the inputting and accessing of consistent and common data concerning population trends, health service activity, referral patterns, usage and systems of booking hospital beds etc.

As part of the evolutionary development of the network, FHSAs and GPs communicate through more direct day-to-day working contact. More practice population health needs information is routinely provided by GPs. Work has yet to be done in setting up information systems for compatibility with Health Authorities. There is continuing emphasis being placed on FHSAs to develop information systems for the general monitoring and management of the Family Health Services, for monitoring GP performance, and for monitoring drug prescribing procedures. FHSAs are taking increasing responsibility for gathering information on morbidity patterns and more specifically regarding the shifting of patients between GPs.

Computerisation of general practices has been demonstrated as essential for collection and retrieval of District level health information. FHSAs have established local area networks, advising GPs on the appropriate hardware and software, and generally offering advice on the day-to-day workings and value of health information systems. Since annual reports from GP practices are best based on computerised records, the FHSAs have a crucial role in supporting GPs in data collection and utilisation.

The real challenge for FHSAs continues to be improvement of the quality of data collected, the more effective usage of valuable data already held, and in their own ability to properly receive and use information from the GP reports.

When considering the discussion above, concerning essential requirement for a comprehensive health care system based on the principles of primary health care, FHSAs have been encouraged to see their information needs in terms of their responsibility to review:

- service activity, skill and equipment profile;

- morbidity and mortality;

- referral patterns and prescribing procedures;

- surveillance and health promotion to reduce 'potentially avoidable deaths';

- general trend in consumer need;

- cash-limited and non-cash-limited expenditure;

- pharmaceutical supervision and support for groups with special needs.

The above information and FHSA review is locally based, focussing on identifiable consumer or patient grouping within an established geographical area and emphasises the key role of the general practitioner as the key figure in making PHC work at the ground floor. FHSAs' 'critical success factors' are compatible with those required for the effective collection and usage of information for PHC impact in that FHSAs are required to:

• understand trends in consumer need;

• match service delivery with consumer need;

• develop effective framework and systems of information;

• develop mechanisms to influence suppliers and consumers;

• develop all the ingredients required for effective and responsive FHSA management.

For FHSAs, therefore, the NHS reforms put an emphasis on the value and importance of FHSA population databases for purposes of patient registration, screening and service planning. Comprehensive health provision must be based on a consistent database which ought to be seen in the context of the NHS strategic framework concerning input and access to common data which is exchanged and shared between FHSAs, GPs and Health Authorities. Generally, then, the challenge for FHSAs is to collaborate with DHAs encouraging them to share information particularly with regard to morbidity and mortality statistics, to share collection resources, for effective usage of information as a management tool and for integrated service delivery.

FHSAs have the responsibility to identify what sort of information is required, how comprehensive ought that information to be, what would be the methods of collection and who/which sectors would be involved and have access to a comprehensive District-based health profile from which FHSAs could develop a comprehensive health index for effective and efficient health service planning and delivery.

In a complex health service system, such as we have in the UK, information has often been either inaccurate or non-representative of population health trends or has been collected in inconsistent forms, rendering it incompatible with similar health information independently collected and analysed by a whole range of different health professionals and sectors appropriate to health service delivery. FHSAs, therefore, are working to create an accurate detailed local database and system for efficient updating of that information, as well as to motivate and activate health workers at all levels to compare data sets.

The major concern of FHSAs is to develop collaborative information for service delivery, particularly by integrating computerised patient records with DHA screening programmes, as in the example of the DHA's comprehensive cervical cancer screening programme, whilst maintaining confidential access to, and emphasising, analysis and effective use of efficiently collected relevant patient information for comprehensive primary health care.

Inter-sectoral collaboration is essential to the FHSAs to reduce duplication of information. DHAs, GPs, social services and NHS

Trusts should be encouraged to pool information with FHSAs to enable appropriate evaluation and dissemination of health indicators. The current reluctance of various sectors, both professional and corporate, to release their data undermines this development.

FHSAs, information and community participation

The NHS reforms highlight the responsibility for FHSAs to ensure community involvement in the continuing identification of health issues, problems and needs, as a basis for broad integrated PHC programming, and that the two major means by which that can be achieved could be through:

1. the use of consumer surveys, where FHSAs need to ensure that the views of the public are obtained, and taken into account, by arranging, from time to time, for consumer surveys to be undertaken in relation to representative samples of the population served; and

2. developing means for consumer access, where FHSAs ensure that consumers have readier access to much more information about the family health services provided – a basis for an increase in fair and open competition between FHS providers and as bases for setting performance-level indicators for purposes of determining providers' remuneration-against-performance.

In order for FHSAs to be the instigators and catalysts in the transition from a health service which is a reactive illness-treating service to being a pro-active health-promoting service, they are working to create an environment whereby consumers are well informed and therefore able to exercise the widest range of appropriate choice to suit their needs. It is essential that the general public be involved and have some input into the planning process for Family Health Services.

Information needs of patients

FHSAs certainly are publicising information concerned with new regulations so that the general public are, first of all, informed that it is possible to change doctors. FHSAs need to make sure that local up-to-date information systems are in public places for public access, and local directories will give a range of information about GP services, properly updated to detail relevant and accurate local information. All practices are encouraged to inform the consumer of all issues concerned in the practice to enable a more informed choice by means of individual leaflets grouped into small information area packs and possibly available through such places as libraries and other well-attended public places and distributed by other agencies such as community health councils, etc. All this will have the effect of raising the profile of FHSAs in comparison with the relatively anonymous Family Practitioner Committees.

Generally, then, the FHSAs have an increasing and up-to-date body of data that can be made public in a time when there is already an increasing trend for patients to seek more information before choosing their GP. FHSAs encourage practices to conduct patient-sensitive surveys, the results of which are fed back through discussions between FHSAs and GPs, and used to achieve identifiable and agreed upon improvements to the service. The sharing of experiences of different FHSAs, as progressive practices, is already being made available. These are the results of well-conducted, professionally sound and fully credible surveys and highlight improvements that patients would like to see. FHSAs should encourage this practice to be comprehensively adopted.

Finally, annual practice reports offer patients valuable information about the working of their practices and enable the public to compare the service offered by a range of practices. Patient participation groups, though fostered by the Royal College of General Practitioners, have had little impact, since, as will be discussed later, much local effort is required to set them up and they need the support of GPs who, increasingly, are feeling threatened by both government and local community scrutiny.

What is clear is that FHSAs need to develop streamlined methods by which the working population can be informed and consulted regarding their own health issues by the service being taken to the public with an objective in mind to develop a sophisticated level of community preferences in collaboration with the general practitioners.

The introduction of any health programme or health system has to reflect judgments about the health needs of people living in a certain geographically defined area and, therefore, must reflect decisions to act upon those needs. Needs assessment can be made by professionals using their training and past experience, or by utilising experienced social surveyors etc, to project possible problems or carry out surveys in order to plan actions. FHSAs have already begun to follow this professional-oriented style of assessment, as reflected in the statements above concerning their interpretation of legislative and policy requirements. Professional assessment alone, by definition, migrates against community participation and involvement in expressing needs to which the health service needs to respond. The FHS approach and action from the outset must prioritise the involvement of community members in research and analysis and certain issues and questions need to be raised, therefore, in order for the health service to be truly consumer oriented and most effectively responsive to the public's primary health care needs.

The FHSA approach can already be seen to be prioritising health service and health service professional needs over health needs. Neither FHSAs nor the NHS and Community Care Act adequately address the need for people in the community to have a role in conducting the needs assessments and in analysing community health needs.

When surveys are seen as essential to assessing a community's health requirements, there is no suggestion that the public and their representatives will contribute to the designing and conducting of the surveys. FHSAs have a responsibility to ensure that surveys are not merely used to get information but also to initiate an environment for discussion with the various possible beneficiaries and, with that in mind potential beneficiaries ought also to be involved in analysing the results of surveys and thus encouraged to be involved in future planning and programming.

For primary health care to have any impact on the public, the community, as the beneficiaries of the health service, have therefore, to have an increasingly strengthened role in decision-making about all aspects of the PHC programme and therefore, increasingly, the needs assessment would need to include various representatives from the wide range of possible beneficiaries for which the health programme was designed and which the health system is meant to serve.

Implications for future primary health care

FHSAs will need, from the outset, to ensure that information gathering and usage reflects not a professionally oriented health service for itself, but a people-oriented service which attempts to maximise the potential for individuals and communities to enhance their health status.

FHSAs and management for PHC

The NHS reforms emphasise that FHSAs need to be responsible for the planning and management of broad integrated PHC programmes and services which, in turn, ought to be based on identified community health issues, problems and needs, and particularly, FHSAs need to play an active role in planning the organisation and development of PHC services. Their strengthened and enhanced planning and management role, for efficient and effective service, particularly, emphasises administering arrangements for the level and quality of provision for the general medical services (ie family doctors, dentists, pharmacists, opticians) and for monitoring an enforcement of those service standards.

For FHSAs, the PHC White Paper emphasises a narrower (though valuable) concept of 'monitoring performance', ie that FHSAs will enhance their capacity to manage FH services by utilising output measures and performance indicators for the services, chiefly by referring to practices' annual report submissions to monitor more closely the level and quality of service provision. Further, their management of part-time general dental practice advisers (contracted to FHSAs) who would collaborate with the dental reference officers.

They will be required to exercise a leadership role in securing/ developing more safe, effective and economic drug prescribing, particularly by encouraging the development of repeat prescribing control systems, practice formularies, and other measures to improve cost-effectiveness, and by monitoring individual doctors' prescribing, and supervising supply and safe-keeping of medicines in residential homes. They have a responsibility also to develop the concept of PHC teams across, and at every level of, the PHC programme, for example, through practice team development where their responsibility is for the funding and development of practice teams (including encouraging the establishment of group practices).

FHSAs also have responsibility for financial management of resource allocation, particularly in the context of the NHS and Community Care Act requirements that extra government resources will be allocated where they are most needed and that the exact amount for each of the relevant health services will depend on the outcome of negotiations with the professions concerned. The FHSAs have an obvious role to play here in managing those negotiations and arrangements for allocation, particularly for those who contribute to the provision of primary health care services.

Essentially, the Government, through the NHS and Community Care Act, has sought to devolve to FHSAs as many powers of decision as are consistent with Government's responsibilities to Parliament and its overall responsibility for managing the NHS. At the operational level there are three major areas of management responsibility for FHSAs:

1. managing the GP contract;

2. overseeing GP prescribing; and

3. managing financial resources.

Managing the GP contract

FHSAs' key purpose is to provide quality family doctor services for their residents within the framework of the new GP contract. This entails the FHSAs having a vision of the future which sees health services meeting the requirements of the served community, the development of an effective policy framework out of those needs, ensuring that the profession is motivated to that end and not de-motivated through the shift in power bases suggested in the White Papers. FHSAs have been charged with administering a practical approach in applying the contract for the benefit of the patient and therefore that the spirit of the contract is carried through and they therefore need to develop basic performance indicators which enable evaluation of the health services in accordance with patient needs. There is, therefore, a promise of a huge cultural change within the NHS which affects, more than most, the general practitioner services, and the FHSAs have to develop a strategy for coping with that shift as well as being sensitive and pro-active to the changing relationships between health services (and particularly the DHAs) and the social services. FHSAs' supporting role to GPs, at least in the first instance cannot be emphasised too much. At the same time, they have a responsibility for creating an environment whereby the present vast differences in styles of general practices are minimised, where GPs are encouraged to deliver high-quality services, consistent with their peers, and nurturing of new relationships by FHSAs based on mutual understanding and respect of each other's position will be crucial to the GPs effectively carrying through the contract for maximum PHC impact. It is important that the new contract is not merely seen as a new way of paying GPs but that it is a means of ensuring that standards are raised and maintained and that doctors are more available and more accountable to both their patients and to the FHSAs. Specific details of the working of the GP contract are discussed elsewhere in this volume. However, successful management of the GP contract is the issue here and to do so FHSAs must have:

- clear aims and objectives and a programme of activities to support them;

- local policy and local criteria clearly laid down;

- positive decision-making procedures;

- determination to use the contract wisely to develop services and meet local needs;

- courage to grasp opportunities presented for change and streamlining of contractual implications;

- a firm, consistent but understanding management style which matches the local situation.

This requires FHSAs to involve GPs and the local medical committee from the outset, to use medical advisers, to consider policies of other FHSAs, nationally and locally, to clarify policies so that they are well known and understood by all, to make public those policies using all manner of media. Above all, FHSAs need to use the contract to raise standards and to target poor practices and disadvantaged areas, and that will require expert leadership on behalf of the FHSAs to get their message across to the GPs, using different approaches, according to the motivation, commitment and competence of the GP to best meet FHSA requirements and therefore to best serve the community.

The new contract will give FHSAs the opportunity to encourage or discourage single-handed or group practices. It will enable them to change the balance of care between the FHSA and the DHA. It will enable the FHSA to widen people's choice of services and to develop new and improved services.

It is essential, therefore, that the FHSA have a constructive and positive relationship with both the GPs and the local medical councils, particularly since the NHS reforms emphases are on the surgery being the place where PHC will happen. Thus FHSAs must show flexibility in interpreting the contract, and in interpreting the demands of the regulations concerning implementation of the contract. Consistent management of their dealing with GPs and the establishment of an ongoing two-way communication process will all enhance the FHSAs potential to carry through an essential determination to use the contract to achieve the agreed objective, which must be to enhance the health status of the local served community.

Crucial to the FHSA managerial service is that they have a sense of direction where they develop mission statements, set objectives, plan strategically in order to win the confidence of GPs. GPs, of course, ought to be included in the policy-making/decision-making process particularly to alleviate concerns over appropriateness of service, and so that policies are practice/situation specific. Within FHSAs, it will be crucial to get the decision-making process clear to everyone, especially by encouraging FHSAs personnel to think MBO (management by objectives). And which particularly emphasises a crucial area to the success of FHSAs, how to actually think seriously about making decisions now for immediate action (and even implementation), whilst explaining and making it clear that objectives/policies may change over time according to the needs of the community and to the needs of the GPs.

GP prescribing

Principles laid down in the NHS reforms broadly affect prescribing policies and practices. The primary health care White Paper *Promoting Better Health* emphasises the FHSAs leadership role in implementing such policies and practice; that they encourage a local focus for discussion concerning the policies, practices; that they consider particularly the issues of repeat prescribing and monitor practice formularies, generally monitoring individual doctors' prescribing and enabling the situation whereby people may seek independent medical advice.

The NHS and Community Care Act puts great emphasis on value-for-money/accountability whereby the RHA will set a prescribing budget for each FHSA, where FHSAs set indicative budgets for each practice under their auspices, and where FHSAs monitor the prescribing patterns of those practices.

Out of that, FHSAs will be able to assess variations between practices and make decisions ranging from doing nothing, should current practice costs be justified, give advice through the medical adviser, offer the case of the particular practice for peer review, or sanction inappropriate prescribing as a last resort. As a result, FHSAs ought to be able to collate ongoing information on good prescribing practice and disseminate that amongst all practices under their auspices as a comparative and motivational tool.

Generally, then, the FHSAs have a responsibility for encouraging good prescribing practice, disseminating prescribing information, encouraging practice formulary, monitoring individual practice pre-scribing, have continual discussions with DHAs concerning prescribing, negotiate the FHSA prescribing budget, set practices' indicative budgets and develop ideas for dealing with variations in practices. The FHSAs have a valuable enabler in the medical adviser, particularly to give internal advice to the general manager and the committee and to give advice to practices. The IMA can valuably interpret information to allow good prescribing to flourish and enable the patient to get the medication he or she needs, the GPs to understand data and improve their prescribing practice, the general manager to stay well informed and the RHA and DoH to continually monitor needs of the FHSA 'patch' continually and clearly.

Managing financial resources and cash limits

The introduction of cash-limited practice staff and premises funding, provided that adequate funds are made available, could provide an opportunity for FHSAs to channel funds into practices where they are most needed and also to target new initiatives, particularly those which approach the achievement of the concept of primary health care in practice, and which have perhaps not been given priority attention in the past. FHSAs will need a framework for managing these funds which will involve identifying and targeting of community health need, appropriate distribution and location of service, developing alliances with Local Authorities and DHAs to make maximum use of staff and premises, developing a feedback mechanism from the medical audit, developing practices which are under-resourced, and generally enhancing primary health care and community care teamwork.

FHSAs will need, therefore, to get their information and accounting systems in order and, from there, map out and start the processes of bidding, evaluation, agreement and allocation. Obviously, continued dialogue with practice staff will need to be maintained together with informal reviews of the staffing in some practices, the funding of selective developments or initiatives and the comparing of job descriptions and pay across the FHSA 'patch'.

All the above, of course, will depend on the FHSAs having developed a clear-sighted view of what the local population need is, which will provide the basis and framework from which the FHSA business plan is developed. From this, FHSAs will need to be closely involved in developing practice business plans, meet local population need and to increase the GP awareness of cost improvement and income generation. The FHSA will therefore be in the position of making cost-effectiveness analysis, therefore monitoring financial resources as practice staff funds become limited.

FHSAs will have the task to both encourage and persuade GPs to improve practice services, facilities and premises. They will need to develop a system of being informed in advance of what GPs' plans

are, if effective use is to be made of cash limited funds and bids made
to regions for future funding. The FHSA will need to review GPs'
plans, which ought to be backed with realistic information, and will
need to be clear how cash-limited funds are allocated between staff
and premises. The FHSA should therefore publicise criteria and plans
for cash-limited funds so that all parties (GPs, RHAs, DHAs and the
DoH) are aware of these and plan accordingly. The plans need to have
some flexibility to take account of the varying needs of a 'FHSA patch'
and also unexpected situations. Of course, FHSAs need to work within
criteria and plans and their decision should not be second-guessed by
way of an appeal system. This would make nonsense of cash-limiting
and of the FHSAs new management role in relation to the family doctor
service. Moreover, it would cause uncertainty and delays for GPs, both
those appealing and their colleagues.

All this suggests a substantial role for FHSAs in the management of
financial resources on the side of cost-effectiveness of services being
seen in the context of fairly strict cash limits for general practices.

FHSAs, management and inter-sectoral collaboration

The NHS reforms emphasise that FHSAs enhance collaboration
between the relevant sectors (statutory and voluntary bodies and
organisations) to work together, to effectively maximise their resources
in the interests of patient care, particularly where the policies of one
agency have impact on the services provided by another. It is suggested
that FHSAs in England and Wales could appropriately apply, or adopt,
principles of district-level collaboration and teamwork as highlighted in
the example of Scotland where responsibility for the administration for
family practitioner services is undertaken by 15 health boards and the
Common Service Agency. This integration, within one administrative
organisation, of all hospital, community and primary health care services
is the most appropriate administrative machinery for Scotland given the
scale of the NHS and the distribution of population served by each
health board, and could be administered by FHSAs.

The overall aim is therefore for relevant sectors within the PHC
programme as a whole to collaborate to ensure that the use of health
service resources achieves the maximum benefit for the public and that
services are used to ensure quality of care in a cost-effective way through
joint consultative planning, development and management of efficient
and effective (appropriate) referral between levels of service delivery.
It goes without saying that essential to all this will also be maximum
inter-professional sharing and exchange of appropriate objective advice
and guidance to support effective implementation of the management
function. For example, FHSAs' access to independent medical advice
will be essential for carrying out their leadership function and role in
developing more safe, effective and economic drug prescribing.

Collaboration between FHS and DHAs is vital. A number of areas of necessary overlap are listed below as illustrative of this inter-locking:

- assessing local health needs, where joint population profile data needs to be gathered, where views of users need to be obtained via consumer surveys. GPs, voluntary organisations and such bodies as CHCs and statutory agencies, or in order to identify unmet needs on which the operational objective of the service must be based;

- appraisal of service options which needs to include a critical examination of problems with current patterns of service and issues arising from the medical and nursing audit, identification of options for change for the more effective forms of treatment, appropriate distribution of care across hospital and community and responsibility across DHA and FHSA, and concerning preferred referral patterns of GPs. The joint decision-making process on judging priorities, with the DHA being required to ensure that preferred serviced development plans are consistent with FHSA and other local developments, would be an essential final part of this appraisal;

- both bodies of course would be responsible for the monitoring of services and health and particularly in evaluation changes in health status of the local population and effectiveness of providers of the service.

For this collaboration to work, management issues will particularly have, initially at least, to concentrate on, for example: the management of conflict between the FHSAs and DHAs and the tensions for a struggle over power bases in the control of health services; FHSAs have to improve their data bases in order to establish credibility with DHAs as a prerequisite for improved joint service planning. Of course, liaison between the two and other organisations will be inevitable and essential in order to develop some consistency in collection, and to maximise the use of available information. The FHSAs will, therefore, need to develop their negotiating skills to a reasonably sophisticated level in order to make collaboration effective at both the practical and policy-making levels.

Critical issues and concerns

For primary health care to have impact by means of a comprehensive district-based health service, collaboration at, and between, all levels of the system, from the more senior decision-makers through to professionals and all health related groups, is essential. This collaboration should be both based on, and should encourage, participation of the professionals in the decision-making process so that there is local ownership between professionals and local people.

Inter-sectoral collaboration is essential for the development of a quality assurance monitoring system whereby 'critical success factors' need to be consistent for all sectors involved. The FHSAs, as the coordinating agency for PHC, need to have time and support to minimise vested interest amongst definitions by separate sectors of how they can successfully perform, to therefore reduce multi-dimensional confusion by harnessing vested interests for a consistent PHC vision and set of achievable objectives for the future.

It is essential then that the FHSAs and senior health managers see their leadership role in terms of that which is required in the specific situation of the district, whereby collaboration and participation with other professionals and other sectors, as well as appropriate delegation of authority for decision-making processes to those individuals and sectors, is practised alongside the need to make central government policy workable. Often the failure of PHC programmes has been explained in terms of PHC leaders' obsession with the latter, and what is prescribed in the NHS and Community Services Act might encourage FHSAs to take that very directive line for short-term quantifiable success, but which may mitigate against long-term impact on the health service.

It goes without saying that a priority for FHS ought to be to encourage real district-level PHC teams, reducing the obsession with professional hierarchies as managerial structure for PHC impact, for consistent-integrated decision-making and policy formulation. The FHS's major role here would be to reduce the inertia caused from dual loyalties of professionals to their hierarchical structures and to the PHC teams, and partly encouraged by the competitive spirit of the NHS reforms where professional groups can even more clearly be in conflict over scarce resources and services. Financial incentives, salary structures and a variety of conditions of service, being encouraged as motivational tools, can mitigate against genuine and effective team working. Agreed goals and objectives for disparate populations can only be borne out of district-level PHC teamwork, whereas the NHS reforms suggest that national health needs, and therefore service goals and objectives, are consistent and can be achieved through individual professionals (particularly general practitioners) and through creation of an environment whereby individuals, who ought to be sensitive to, and be working towards, the achievement of local health service success, compete with each other for their own personal professional success.

The NHS reforms' provisions for medical education hint at the retraining of doctors to manage rather than dominate (on clinical status grounds) district health teams. This exacerbates the feeling of resentment from other professionals and leads to ineffective usage of professional skills and knowledge. Government policy does not go far enough to suggest training of DMOs in the essential managerial skills to handle contradictions between their position as clinical practitioners and district health leadership nor between their roles as district health committee member and PHC team member, etc.

It is clear from the White Papers that cost-effectiveness reviews will take place, in terms of the whole resource allocation policy laid down by central government. This could serve to evaluate performance of specific Districts, easily manageable under the auspices of particular FHSs, but again the interpretation of national policy through to local implementation has taken on the character of individual health professionals and individual specialist services being evaluated in term of their cost-effectiveness. This mitigates against essential collaboration between all sectors at the District level, again where competition over scarce resources forms the basis of evaluation of performance rather than in terms of collaborative District-level PHC/health service impact.

Central government may be better served to identify or encourage specific local pilot projects, which target their PHC priority action and which are based on inter-sectoral involvement and collaboration, evaluating success according to a collective effort for health organisation output and health impact, and which promote that 'mode' (emphasising its use if adapted specifically to suit Districts' unique situations) and therefore place, in the public eye, an emphasis on the different sectors discussed above working together under the scrutiny and direction of the FHSA.

Finally, inter-sectoral collaboration emphasises the value of all involved in the development of the local health potential. Collaboration motivates individuals by offering a major incentive of empowering people at the District level, community and professionals alike, as inputs to the decision-making and action required in relation to their own health needs. This tangible feedback of input by the community and professionals serves to overcome de-motivating aspects of a hierarchical health structure, encouraged, it has to be said, by policy deliberation out of central government, and which takes on the form of a lack of status and power over the decision-making process for a most inconsistent system for financial rewards which tend to be aimed anyway at senior people in the health service hierarchy, and threats of a lowering in conditions of employment and therefore in security for the majority of health workers.

FHSAs are presented here with an ideal opportunity to orchestrate networks linking all levels of government, health profit and Community to form an effective multi-dimensional communication system to enhance health performances, management performance and the quality of collaboration and teamwork. Inter-sectoral collaboration best enables FHSAs to translate government policy into appropriate implementation and impact of PHC provision according to local needs and through the effort of 'locally sensitive' health professionals and local community.

Conclusion

Primary health care is more than a set of services or programmes delivered as part of National Health Service provision. It incorporates the necessity for change, requiring changes in conceptualising health and health care and therefore changes in ways of thinking about health and health provision.

Implementing PHC requires appreciation of development of a process which questions, and which calls for, wide-ranging changes in established systems and institutions, pertinent to communities and their development. The concept of PHC has at its core, an acceptance that individuals, families and communities can and do take the major responsibility for their own health. Health professionals and health systems need to take on the role of assisting and supporting this process.

Central to the effectiveness of FHSAs in this role, therefore, would be the development of methods and techniques for working with communities, emphasising that each community has its own particular needs, in order to satisfy a PHC prerequisite that a 'bottom-up' approach for the identification of needs and for the setting of targets be adhered to. These needs and targets would, in turn, determine FHSAs, and health organisations under their auspices, 'top-down' actions and decisions. The message here would be that, via FHSAs, the health system and its related organisation would need to set their objectives and determine their activities in relation to those expressed by the communities which they serve. Such a working style necessitates a continuing process of dialogue, popular consultation, organisational adapting and change, all highlighted in the above discussion.

Training FHSAs for PHC in the UK

Management training initiatives will need to be developed through appropriate forums whereby FHSA managers can examine positive and realistic approaches to tackling their formidable set of responsibilities. They will need to be supported in identifying and examining their role and function in identifying priorities and keeping performance targets for the FHSA, in considering the most effective utilisation of resources in pursuit of these priorities and, through a supportive learning environment, would be encouraged to focus on specific topics and issues particularly pertinent to their own FHSA and specially in the context of the needs and demand of primary health care development in their district(s).

If FHSAs are to be the pioneers and leaders in implementing the change required for effective PHC in the UK, the managers will require support in:

- determining their 'critical success factors', through mission develop-ment and objective-setting for strategic policy formulation towards development of performance indicators for monitoring the achieve-ment of FHSA/PHC targets;

- developing staff and PHC professionals for policy implementation, especially through the announcement of their leadership skills, management style and decision-making expertise;

- managing conflict, through gaining contractor confidence, and 'getting things done' through the GP contract, through GP indicative prescribing and through practice funding;

- developing a working strategy for inter-sectoral collaboration, in order to enhance the development of practical working relationships with RHAs, DHAs, Local Authorities, local medical committees, GPs, directors of public health, and all sectors essential for effective family health/PHC services;

- creating mechanisms for a community-oriented service and community consultation through an appreciation of, and skills in, community participation/involvement as a vehicle for effective PHC services.

All the above has been an attempt to constructively debate the implications of the NHS reforms for the improvement of primary health care in the UK, giving particular attention to the role of the new family health service authorities in developing local health services which meet with the principles of primary health care. However they also meet with the governments key objectives, ie:

- to enable clearer priorities to be set for family health services in relation to the rest of the health service;

- to raise standards of care;

- to promote health and prevent illness;

- to improve value for money in the health service;

- to make services more responsive to the consumer;

- to give patients the widest range of choice in obtaining high quality primary care services.

References

Alma Ata Declaration, Section VII-4.
Alma Ata Declaration, Section VII-5.
Alma Ata Declaration, Section VII-6.
DHSS (1987) *Promoting Better Health* Cmd 249, HMSO, London.
DHSS (1989) *Caring for People* Cmd 555, White Paper, November 1989, HMSO, London.
DoH (1989) *Working for Patients* White Paper, HMSO, London.
DoH (1991) *The Health of the Nation* HMSO, London.
Ebrahim, GJ and Ranken, JP (1988) *Primary Health Care: Reorienting Organisational Support* Macmillan, London.
National Health Service and Community Care Act, 1990 HMSO, London.
Nordic School of Public Health (1984) *Methods and Experience in Planning for Health: Inter-sectoral Action for Health* Report NHV 1984:2, NSPH, Goteburg, Sweden.

Oakley, P (1989) *Community Involvement in Health Development: an Examination of the Critical Issues* 51-7 World Health Organisation, Geneva.

Report No: EUR/ICP/PHC 1399/g51, WHOEURO, Copenagen *Social Science and Medicine* (1988) **26**, 9, 877-971, Pergamon Press, Oxford.

Society for Family Practitioner Committees/NHSTA/DoH (1990) *Promoting Better Health and the GP Contract* Jan, Society for FPCs, London.

WHO (1978) *Final report of the international conference on primary health care* Alma Ata, USSR, Sept 6–12, 1978. World Health Organisation, Geneva.

WHO (1987) *Hospitals and health for all* Technical Report Series No: 744, World Health Organisation, Geneva.

WHO (1987) *Interaction between health and social services and the public in the provision of health care* Report on a WHO Working Group, Granada, Spain, 16–20 November, 1987. Report No: WHO/EUR/PHC 330, WHO, Copenhagen.

WHO (1988) *Strengthening ministries of health for primary health care* Technical Report Series 766, World Health Organisation, Geneva.

WHO (1989a) *District health systems in action – ten years after Alma Ata – experiences and future directions* Report on a workshop, Neubrandenburg, GDR, 5–9 December 1988.

WHO (1989b) *Management of Human Resources for Health* Technical Report Series 783, World Health Organisation, Geneva.

10 General practice – a force for change

Andrew Willis

Introduction

This chapter considers some of the implications of the NHS reforms for general practice. It begins with a historical sketch of major influences for change that have taken place, and the profession's response to them. It then goes on to consider some of the key elements of the new, expanding role for general practice within the NHS. The chapter closes by describing what are seen as desirable characteristics of strategies intended both to maximise benefits obtained from the reforms, and to minimise any disadvantages.

Historical background

The NHS reforms of 1989/91 had several components, including major changes in the general practitioner's contract (DoH 1989a) as well as the implementation of the White Paper *Working for Patients*. The contractual changes in fact stemmed from a previous White Paper (DoH 1988) and there have been other relevant documents arising from both *Working for Patients* and The National Health Service and Community Care Act 1990. For convenience all of these will here be referred to collectively as the reforms.

Prior to 1989 there were five events that had particularly fundamental significance for future general practice. These were The National Insurance Act of 1911, the formation of The National Health Service in 1948, the foundation of The Royal College of General Practitioners in 1952, the Charter for The Family Doctor Service, which was constructed in 1965, and the availability of microcomputers from the late 1970s. Of these the first was the most important, for the National Insurance Act laid the foundation stones of general practice by introducing the registered list of patients, referral system, capitation payments, and the self-employed status of the GP. As Richards observes, once these key elements had been created the formation of the NHS in 1948 merely represented their formalisation and development (Richards 1988). The Royal College of General Practitioners has led the fields of research, education and the development of information systems, and accordingly raised the standing and credibility of general practice. For example, for many years prior to the reforms it had been undertaking research into improving quality within general practice (Buck *et al.* 1974; Irvine 1983, RCGP 1985a, b, Buckley 1989). The advent of commercially available microcomputers heralded the most significant change in clinical records since 1911, though the true potential of computer technology has only in recent years been explored on the required scale.

Nonetheless it was the action in 1965 of the General Medical Services Committee (GMSC) of the British Medical Association (BMA) that had the greater initial effect on the development of general practice. At a time of 'profound malaise and disorder within general practice' (BMJ 1965) members of that committee produced a Charter for the Family Doctor Service that called for assistance with obtaining appropriate practice premises, the attachment of community staff to practices, support for post-graduate education, help with the employment of receptionists and secretaries, the reduction of the average list size to 2000 patients and trials of different methods of payment for GPs. As a result of the Charter a new contract was negotiated by the GMSC, the result being the birth of modern general practice with embryonic Primary Health Care Teams working from appropriate premises. Remarkably, in practical terms the contract placed no restrictions upon the level of resources available, but provided inadequate motivation for most practices to alter their behaviour to make good use of them. The profession's failure to seize that opportunity for development proved to be the seed-corn for the Government's move, some 23 years later, to introduce a further, more prescriptive, contract (DoH 1988, DoH 1989a).

Conversely the current reforms provide motivation for behavioural change (albeit some of it coercive) but relatively few additional resources. Partly because of the internal market, clinicians from primary and secondary care are now working together to improve local services in a way that has not happened before.

By one method or another GPs and hospital clinicians are being made accountable for their expenditure and so the thrust for cost effectiveness is supported. Whether through fundholding or other means purchasing is increasingly concerned with quality, value for money, and sensitivity to the needs of local communities and individual patients. That the effect appears to pass responsibility for rationing NHS resources from the Government to the medical profession is politically fortunate. One effect of purchasers considering cost effectiveness will be a long needed shift of resources away from the acute hospital sector into the community. This imbalance and need is particularly well illustrated by Sir Bernard Tomlinson in relation to Central London (Tomlinson 1992).

The Royal Commission into the NHS (Merrison 1979) set out broad aims for the NHS which included:

- equality of entitlement;
- the provision of a broad range of services of a high standard;
- a service that is free at the time of use;
- a service that satisfies the reasonable expectations of its users;
- a service that remains a national service responsive to local needs.

It seems reasonable to believe that these aims for the NHS remain the 'reasonable expectations of its users' and the ones inherent in most people's understanding of the remark 'the NHS is safe in our hands', a remark unaccompanied by any alternative definition of the service it refers to (Fowler 1991). Thus for at least two reasons the aims expressed by Merrison are central to any discussion of the reforms and general practice. First, they describe the fundamental characteristics of the NHS as understood by the public. Second, they illustrate how the NHS is essentially different from most other health care systems, and, importantly, from that in the USA, to which favourable parallels have been drawn by those advocating some aspects of the reforms. The USA has no pretensions to providing resident populations with equality of entitlement to a comprehensive health service funded largely out of taxation. Even American Health Maintenance Organisations (HMOs) do not have such a broad remit for their focussed, catchment populations as does the NHS for its non-discretionary, resident ones. In the wake of the reforms the goal of equality of entitlement related to clinical need will not always be practical where priorities differ amongst purchasers representing different elements of a District's population. However at least the overall allocation of resources to populations should be determined equitably and purchasing priorities then decided by as wide and representative a body of local opinion as possible (NHSME 1992).

Two conclusions arise from this brief historical review. First, it illustrates how the medical profession tends to respond in a reactionary manner to proposed change, but is pragmatically constructive in implementing changes once these are established. While the 1911 Act and the negotiations at the time of the Charter were associated with major hostility from the profession towards the Government, with threats of mass resignation on both occasions, three of the major landmarks, the College, the Charter itself, and the development of microcomputer systems were the result of initiatives by the profession in response to its inappropriate working conditions or information systems. Second, it may be concluded that in order to bring about beneficial change the profession requires appropriate resources and the motivating forces to make use of them. One is little use without the other. The 1965 contract in effect provided unlimited resources but little motivation. The 1990 reforms provide creative motivation for some aspects of the work, but little more than contractual coercion for others. At the same time they ultimately threaten to restrict resources for all in order to sustain the central theme of cost containment.

The reforms offer general practice many opportunities to help improve the quality and value of services within the NHS. The main threat is their inherent ability to erode some of the aims defined by the Royal Commission. The challenge is to avoid that risk, and to seize the opportunities provided to improve the service in line with those aims. Never before has general practice had such an opportunity to act as a force for change within the Health Service. But never before has it had such an opportunity to divide it and to increase inequity.

What should general practice be doing?

For general practice to bring about effective change requires a clear overall goal, adequate resources, appropriate motivation and effective education. The reforms introduce two additional, objective elements to the aims of the Royal Commission; the need to make the most effective use of finite resources, and the need to raise the quality of services. Together these aims illustrate that no single practice can look upon itself as a solitary entity, as might an American HMO, for each practice remains an integral component of its Health District. The term 'internal market' implies a corporate approach, utilising market forces between the constituent components of an organisation to stimulate efficiency and effectiveness to benefit the organisation as a whole. Within such a market entrepreneurial activity is to be encouraged. However, particularly within a National Health Service, such activity should be sensitive to the legitimate needs of other communities and not permitted to disadvantage them in an inequitable manner. This need for cohesion of services within a District requires emphasis, for the nature of the fundholding scheme in particular may prompt some to underrate its significance.

It is difficult to state what should be done within general practice when few have attempted to define its objectives and fewer still have analysed the overall activity taking place within it. The new contract of 1989 begins to set specific objectives, but before this the GP had only vague, conceptual descriptions for guidance. Hence a statement from The Second European Conference on the Teaching of General Practice, held in Leewenhorst, Netherlands in 1974 concluded: 'The general practitioner is a licensed medical graduate who gives personal, primary and continuing care to individuals, families and a practice population, irrespective of age, sex and illnesses; it is the synthesis of these functions which is unique' (Leewenhorst 1974). Even with the new contract there remains no clear, objective and comprehensive job description, and where attempts are made to include such description, for example with regard to some elements of preventive care, they may be seen as simplistic, of variable medical validity, and as being far from GPs' own experienced perception of the prime functions of their work.

Practices will develop as service businesses, improving both their responsiveness to patient demands and needs, and the quality and range of services they provide. In the past this response and development has been restricted by a system that has failed to motivate practices adequately to raise the quality of their services. A change should be encouraged towards a more reasoned, rational service that seeks to make the best use of available resources to provide:

- effective, demand-sensitive acute services;

- acceptable, cost-effective programmes of preventive procedures of proven benefit;

- and facilities for chronic disease management that are convenient for patients, adequately resourced, and of high quality.

Practices should be encouraged to recognise their responsibility to the evolving local community for medical and social care. Thus they should accept the need to make the most effective use of available resources, both within their own organisations and also with their use of resources shared with other practices. This need also extends to contributing to assessments of needs and outcomes led by the FHSA and DHA, and involving other local voices (NHSME 1992). The search for cost effectiveness will bring pressure to bear upon services of doubtful benefit, but caution is necessary. Numerous surveys of patient opinion demonstrate that intangible characteristics such as time to listen, kindness, accessibility and empathy are deemed to be of great importance (Cartwright and Anderson 1979, Allen 1989). Indeed, as Allen observes, the results of such surveys commonly afford such characteristics higher priority than clinical skills, and in the past they have been an indicator of good general practice. There are dangers in paying too much attention to the credo calling for objective evidence of clinical benefit. To do so is to disregard valued, intangible qualities of carers and caring, and to reduce decision-making to valuing only that which can be measured. A careful balance has to be retained between scientific objectivity, market forces within a service industry, the assessment of needs of populations both large and local, and the humane characteristics of the best carers.

Further, the intention should be for cohesion rather than division between the different groups of health care professionals within a District. Competition should be used to raise standards but not at the expense of increased inequity, poor use of overall resources, or an unnecessarily large shift in the balance of resource usage from clinical services to administration. General practices should be encouraged to respond to the demands of their patient populations whilst at the same time assessing health needs with regard to chronic disease management, preventive medicine and health promotion. Such assessments are inevitably intertwined with those concerning outcomes and resource management. All will involve increasing amounts of work within the practice's own organisation as well as in collaboration with other practices, locality, DHA and FHSA. In this way the cycle of quality assurance will become a fundamental of healthcare provision; the assessment of need prompting appropriate objectives, resource allocations and implementation plans, the outcomes of which are assessed before being amended for greater effect in the light of that experience. Crucially, such a cycle will be informed by advice from specialists in public health medicine, by centres of expertise such as The Cochrane Centre, and by different professions working together on locally agreed objectives. It will be facilitated by the local selection of priorities freeing resources from one activity to be used with greater effect on another, and by increasingly sophisticated techniques for local outcome assessment. Other areas of practice-based data processing inherent in the reforms will involve the administrative farming of the patient list in pursuit of efficient chronic disease management and preventive medicine, and the collection of data to inform the processes of purchasing primary and secondary care. Much of this activity is only feasible within all but small, well motivated practices with the assistance of computers and electronic communications. At the time of writing it would appear that the cost implications of this explosion in clerical activity have yet to be fully appreciated.

Paragraph 1.2 of Working Paper 3, *Working for Patients* (DoH 1989b) sets out the Government's aim to 'offer GPs an opportunity to improve the quality of services on offer to patients, to stimulate hospitals to be more responsive to the needs of GPs and their patients, and to develop their own practices for the benefit of their patients'. Buckley recalls that The New Leewenhorst Group identified three essentials for improving quality; motivation within practices, provision of appropriate resources, and training in necessary skills (Buckley 1989). So far these three key elements of change management have been provided for those within the GP fundholding scheme and there are early signs that they do indeed stimulate change, particularly within the practices themselves. They should now be provided for all practices in order that all patients may benefit from improved services, and that all practices may work together with local health authorities to bring about the integrated, cohesive change needed to ensure improvement in line with the aims established by the Royal Commission, while striving for ever better value for money.

How should it be done?

Initially the most obvious component of the internal market involved secondary care. Somewhat less obvious, and certainly slower to emerge, were the markets in primary care and in purchasing itself. No area of the service is absolved from this shift of responsibility and accountability, nor from the introduction of competition. District

Health Authorities will respond to the market in purchasers or see their authority and negotiating leverage reduce as large numbers of practices turn away from them to become fundholders, or to group within 'Superfunds'. A more constructive way forward is for DHAs to expand the options available by providing a range of mechanisms for GPs to be involved in commissioning and purchasing that is sensitive to their differing, preferred levels of commitment (Morley 1993). In this way all practices within a District, whether fundholders or not, can be affiliated to the overall policies of the FHSA and DHA, working in alliance towards common goals. The level to which DHAs respond to the market in purchasers has a far reaching influence on the future cohesion of services within their Districts.

To a certain extent GPs can select the level of their own participation by deciding whether or not to become fundholders. There have been well publicised examples of pioneering developments by some fundholding practices. In the same way pioneers followed other innovations, such as the Charter of 1965 and the introduction of micro-computers. A lesson from both of those is that in neither case was the behaviour of the extreme pioneers echoed in the subsequent behaviour of the majority until additional incentives were provided. However, neither of them was supported by the weight of political will that has accompanied the reforms, nor by such a blanket assumption of superior quality being applied to those practices employing the latest developments. To equate high quality general practice with fundholding *per se*, and by inference lower quality with non-fundholding, implies that only through fund-holding can the goals be achieved of involving all practices in decisions concerning the setting of local priorities, increasing patient choice and pursuing higher quality services and cost-effectiveness. This is incorrect, and such narrow perceptions reduce the opportunity for more comprehensive and satisfactory solutions to emerge. It is worthy of note that when Enthoven first proposed an internal market for the NHS he made no mention of fundholding for GPs (Enthoven 1985).

Practice management

Norman Fowler considers that the introduction to the NHS of 'modern management' was the Government's greatest achievement in health care in the 1980s (Fowler 1991, p. 198). A considerable benefit of the GPFH scheme is that it has established, *en passant*, effective methods of management within general practice where other initiatives, such as that instigated by the RCGP in 1985, failed to gain wide appeal (RCGP 1985). Given adequate motivation some GPFHs and non-fundholding practices have adopted techniques of quality assurance (Lomas 1990, Irvine 1990) and total quality management (Berwick, Enthoven and Bunker 1992a, 1992b). Such management methods have at their core a recursive process of establishing goals, encouraging and enabling movement towards them, and then assessing progress and outcomes to inform the next planning phase.

This shift to a more structured management style will apply to a greater or lesser extent to all practices and is of greater significance than more widely publicised changes such as imposed involvement in preventive medicine. By encouraging quality assurance within general practice the questioning, objective attitude described over three decades ago by Eimerl (1960), and experienced more recently by GPs attending industrial training courses (Willis 1984), may at last become an accepted component of general practice. This is a major effect of the NHS reforms, setting the management of general practices upon a more professional footing, with quality assurance the driving force for improving quality, accountability and cost-effectiveness.

The implications for the administration of practices are considerable. Some of this activity will be assisted by information technology, including the electronic transfer of information to and from the FHSA and hospitals, but the net effect will remain an increase in work for the practice team. Without appropriate resources and training to support this work morale within practice teams will drop progressively as personnel sink beneath a rising tide of clerical, administrative and managerial activity, and the full potential for development inherent in the reforms will not come to fruition.

The GP as supplier

Practices will increasingly be seen as suppliers of primary care services working under renewable contract to the FHSA, or some form of local commissioning agency that may evolve from these authorities. As purchasers these will increasingly determine the manner in which practices develop, issuing requisite quality standards such as those prepared by Essex Family Health (1992). It is in everyone's interest that practices and FHSAs work closely together, agreeing common goals and ways forward within localities, and minimising the adversarial components of the purchaser–provider relationship. It is of interest that as DHAs at last divest themselves of Directly Managed Units and are freed from bi-polar management to become pure purchasers, some FHSAs are eagerly adopting just such a role for themselves, on the one hand continuing to support practices and on the other becoming purchasers of primary care services.

Acute care

The acute care of general practice remains much as it always has been. In 1960 Spence wrote:

> *The essential unit of medical practice is the occasion when, in the intimacy of the consulting room or sick room, the person who is ill or believes himself to be ill, seeks the advice of a doctor whom he trusts. This is a consultation, and all else in the practice of medicine derives from it.*

(Spence 1960)

It is less the characteristics of the acute consultation that will change, more the manner in which acute care is organised and delivered as a responsive, service business. The Patients' Charter (DoH 1991) indicates the need for greater sensitivity to the demands of patients, and practices will develop the crisp administrative efficiency of commercial service industries whilst at the same time striving to deliver the unhurried intimacy within the consulting room that is described by Spence. Thus the emphasis will be upon using available resources to improve the range, convenience and acceptability to patients of practice procedures and facilities.

Preventive medicine
Before the 1989 contract secondary preventive medicine had little place in a GP's terms of service. Nonetheless a significant number of practices undertook procedures of known benefit either opportunistically or within planned screening programmes. The 1989 contract introduced secondary preventive medicine as a requirement. Some of the procedures selected were of little if any proven clinical value, taking up clinical time when, ironically, the reforms were championing cost-effectiveness. This allowed critics to justifiably ridicule this part of the contract until some of the procedures were withdrawn. More focussed plans for the delivery of preventive care were subsequently drawn up in agreement with the GMSC, though certain elements of these will again be open to challenge (GMSC 1993). Whatever the requirements at any particular time it is clear that the content of preventive medicine will now be driven by external authorities, that those authorities will monitor the effect of their policies, and that an element of remuneration will be linked to satisfactory performance. The delivery of secondary preventive medicine will increasingly become the preserve of practice employed nurses, supported by clerical staff and appropriate clinical computer systems.

Chronic disease management
Ways must be found to enable all practices to work with their purchasers to allow clinical activity to take place where it can most appropriately provide high quality care for the patients for whom it is intended. Clearly where services that have traditionally taken place in the hospital sector are better provided in the community then resources should be moved to allow this to happen, regardless of whether the practice is a fundholder or not. However there are two caveats. First, resource allocations should be equitable, and second, there should be no unacceptable knock-on effect to other services. It is a dubious benefit within a District if the consultant performing an out-reach clinic in one practice leaves junior staff to conduct the main clinic in hospital out-patients. The proper management of those caveats is an important reason for the DHA and FHSA to coordinate the overall health care provision within the District, a responsibility that they alone hold. The effective discharge of that responsibility is assisted by these Authorities

not only having good working relations with themselves but also with a representative body of all local general practices. Further incentives to the structuring of chronic disease management within general practice are also provided within the 1993 arrangements for preventive health care negotiated with the GMSC and referred to above.

While there are advantages in practices organising clinics for specific chronic diseases there are also disadvantages. These should be debated and not swept aside on a wave of simplistic dogma that assumes that if services are moved from hospital to general practice then the format of outpatient clinics should follow as well. Continuity of care is a tradition of general practice much valued by some patients, and particularly by those with chronic diseases. The emerging semi-specialised clinic can break up that continuity of care, and restrict rather than extend the services available to patients. This must be weighed against any technical benefit of sub-specialisation within practice teams. Different practices will arrive at different conclusions but all are likely to be subject to the same contractual pressure to provide chronic disease management clinics. Again, the past variability of practice is being corralled by imposed requirements that seek to raise the standard of relatively poor performers. It would be regrettable if the traditional pragmatism and invention of general practice is diminished in this controlling process. The desired outcome is high quality clinical services. The decision, for example, to only accept for financial reward methods of chronic disease management that utilise clinics requires greater justification than that this is the easiest way for FHSAs to monitor the process, or that this is the way it is done in hospital. FHSAs should exhibit flexibility for different approaches wherever the realistic objective is to offer high quality services. What would happen, for example, if a survey conducted to support a practice's own Patients' Charter, established that patients preferred not to have a clinic structure for the management of chronic diseases, but to see their own doctors within routine consulting sessions?

Social care
At the time of writing the impact of introducing the White Paper *Care in the Community* has yet to be assessed. However in some areas the idea of notional social care budgets attached to individual practices is already being addressed. This is a logical extension of the practice budgets, whether real or notional, introduced by the reforms. With or without social care budgets it is inevitable that social services will interact more closely with general practice, and 'primary health care teams' will presumably evolve into 'primary care teams', including a formal social care component.

The GP as purchaser

Working for Patients describes two alternative methods for involving GPs in the purchasing of secondary care on behalf of their patients. The first is for commissioning and purchasing to be undertaken by the DHA, with the process informed by GP opinion. This has the advantages of centralised coordination of resource utilisation and economies of scale, but may lack sensitivity to the needs of local communities. Such sensitivity is an objective of the reforms and is enabled by the alternative option, the GP fundholding scheme. This voluntary scheme devolves a budget directly from the Regional Health Authority to individual practices, permitting the virement of money between its three elements; those for purchasing secondary care, prescribing and for employing practice staff. It also provides the necessary training in practice management, commissioning, negotiation, and contract management, together with appropriate funding to support additional practice staff and computer systems. It therefore goes a long way to providing the three requirements described by The New Leewenhorst Group as necessary for bringing about change in general practice; resources, motivation, and education (Buckley 1989). The fund can be seen as a budget for the whole of primary care, with the purchasing of secondary care as a mere component of that provision (Colin-Thorne 1991).

Nonetheless the scheme has significant disadvantages, of which its tendency to divisiveness creates some anomalies within a health service aspiring to the aims of the Royal Commission. Furthermore the fund currently only covers about 20 per cent of a practice's expenditure on secondary services. Thus it duplicates rather than replaces DHA purchasing even for GPFHs, creating increased overall administrative expenditure and scope for discordance within the planning of local health care provision. It is too early to judge the effectiveness of the scheme, for GPFHs have been advantaged in various ways to get if off the ground. Perversely it is the small size of GPFHs as purchasers in comparison to DHAs, and their lack of responsibility for a geographical community or Directly Managed Unit (DMU), that has given them leverage within the market that exceeds the proportional size of their funds. It should also be remembered that DHAs were required to avoid 'turbulence' during the first year of the reforms, and maintain a 'steady state' within the market by not moving resources between providers. This may be seen as a remarkable recognition of the potential purchasing power of DHAs working with a large number of practices, particularly when freed of responsibility for DMUs. As Ham observes, under all these circumstances it would indeed be astonishing if fundholders had not been able to bring about improvements in services for their patients (Ham 1993).

Because neither of the two initial options provide an entirely satisfactory solution to the problem of how to involve all GPs in commissioning and purchasing, a range of additional methods have arisen. These were assessed in 1992 within an option appraisal project undertaken by a group of Northampton GPs (NHA 1992). Most consist of some form of centralised purchasing by Health Authorities but with a greater sensitivity in commissioning to the needs of practices, communities and individuals. Some concentrate on the needs of small communities, or localities, involving GPs and other local voices in locality purchasing (Stockport 1992, Ham 1992) Within practice sensitive purchasing (PSP) notional budgets are calculated for each practice and managed by the Health Authority on their behalf, after the practice's purchasing requirements have been established (Tarnowski 1992). Because of economies of scale associated with centralised purchasing, budgets can include a substantially larger percentage of activity than those of the GPFH scheme. A further possibility is for a large number of practices to become fundholders and then pool their administrative efforts within a superfund. The Northampton project concluded that no single method has been developed that accommodates all the requirements for GP involvement in optimising health care within a District. This finding emphasises the need to support and assess prototypes of different methods, and to encourage a variety of solutions to evolve.

Commissioning and purchasing are not the only ways in which GPs can be involved in improving quality and cost-effectiveness of services. A major benefit of the reforms is that they have facilitated discussion between GPs and specialists. While there is now an emphasis on research and development within Regions it has been observed that there is an additional need, perhaps a greater one, to effectively disseminate and apply existing knowledge (HSM 1991). The same Northampton report emphasises the value of what it refers to as speciality liaison groups (SLGs), small focus groups containing representative GPs and specialists from a particular clinical discipline within a District. The aim of SLGs is to find pragmatic ways of making the best use of available resources (NHA 1993). This should be a two-way process, on the one hand with the production of clinical guidelines for general practitioners, and on the other for the meetings to be a forum within which GPs can express their requirements, as direct or indirect purchasers, to their specialist colleagues. This dialogue across the primary and second care interface is an important component of postgraduate education, of maintaining good working relationships between specialists and GPs at a time when the market threatens their division, and of providing an economical mechanism for GPs to convey to consultants the services they require from secondary care.

Conclusion: the need for cohesion and motivation

This chapter set out to consider the reforms as a means of pursuing the aims of the NHS as defined by the Royal Commission. The reforms place emphasis on three matters, improving quality, sensitivity and value for money. They pursue these by devolving decision-making and accountability to the periphery, and by introducing competition through an internal market. In doing so they encourage bottom-up innovation and sensitivity but at the risk of threatening the cohesion of necessary top-down planning and coordination of District policies. The concluding section of the chapter addresses this tension by describing some of the desirable attributes of sustainable District strategies for involving GPs in developing primary and secondary care.

Purchasing
The aim should be to obtain effective GP influence in an economical and equitable manner that can involve all practices in decisions about all, or nearly all, activity. This should minimise fragmentation and administrative overheads whilst being sensitive to the needs of local communities and individuals. Such an aim suggests:

- *Co-ordinated planning at District level* Led by the DHA and FHSA this should involve a democratically elected, representative core group of GPs. The membership of such a group should echo any locality structure used within the District, and contain both GPFHs and non-fundholders. It should have a mandate from the Local Medical Committee to represent the District's practices concerning all purchasing activity other than that negotiated separately, for example by GPFHs or within schemes for locality or practice sensitive purchasing.

- *Professional needs assessment at a community level* This should be based on a locality structure defined around pragmatic clusters of general practices, and involving as wide a pool of local voices as possible. This commissioning activity should be supported by specialists from the District's Department of Public Health.

- *Equitable resource allocations* Differing priorities from different purchasers may lead to variations in access to services, but resource allocations should be determined on an equitable basis.

- *Professional purchasing and contract management* Economies of scale will be available from sharing scarce expertise, whether within consortia of GPFHs, superfunds or Health Authorities acting as purchasing agencies for non-fundholders and non-funded activity.

- *Involvement of clinicians in resource management* Quality assurance within practices inevitably considers the most effective use of resources. Similarly clinicians from primary and secondary care can work together through specialty liaison groups to obtain the best value and quality from the available money.

- *Appropriate motivation to encourage participation and behavioural change* GPs working with the DHA and FHSA on commissioning and purchasing should receive appropriate remuneration. Furthermore information systems should be developed to identify and value all resource use at a practice level, or by locality as an intermediary stage. Already prescribing costs are available at a practice level, and several FHSAs are devolving notional staff budgets to non-fundholders. Once Health Authorities can cost all secondary care

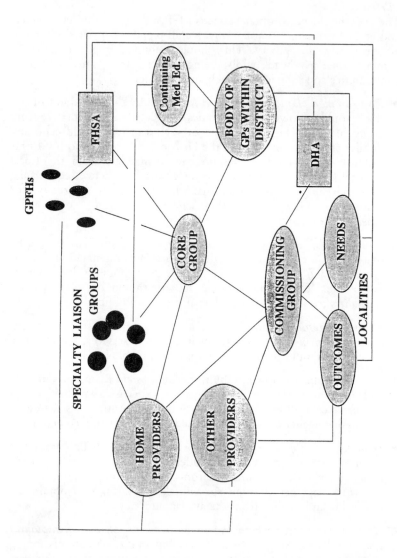

Figure 10.1 Coordinating GP influence on developing primary and secondary care within a District

activity at a practice level the logical end-game of practice sensitive purchasing becomes possible. In addition it permits the additional motivation of virement within the hospital services budget, even if current legislation does not permit transfer of funds between this element of practice expenditure and the FHSA controlled staff and prescribing budgets. Such motivation will allow practices to define their own priorities on behalf of their patients and thereby release resources from certain activities to be used on others with greater effect and relevance.

- *Avoidance of duplication of effort* Multiple purchasers within a District increase administrative overheads in general, including those for providers with an inevitable rise in unit costs. They also weaken the negotiating hand of purchasers.

Providing
Ways must be found for all practices to be offered the resources, motivation and training necessary for their development, with a particular emphasis on management utilising quality assurance. The enhanced role for general practice, promoted by the reforms, has considerable cost implications in terms of developing practice premises, information systems, staffing levels and training. Independent agencies are likely to be developed to facilitate the provision of such training direct to practices. As the move gathers pace to move services from hospitals to the community pragmatic clusters of like-minded practices are likely to emerge to share resources and expertise. Here again there will be value in having a representative group of GPs to maintain a District-wide perspective concerning policy issues and the equitable distribution of resources. This group can either be the LMC, or as proposed earlier an elected core group mandated by the LMC to represent all practices in relation to purchasing. There is considerable merit in the same representative group dealing with both primary and secondary care, as this simplifies the process and facilitates the appropriate placement of services within hospitals and the community.

As FHSAs assume a larger purchasing role locality teams are likely to emerge for the purpose of planning and coordinating local primary and secondary care. These will include GPs, other primary care contractors, local voices, social services, the FHSA and DHA. Priority should be given to finding ways for these teams to avoid becoming bureaucratic, unwieldy, and self-defeating, and to having access to motivating, discretionary funds as described in the previous section.

Strategies that encompass the above points minimise the risks of fragmentation within local medical communities, the development of a multi-tier service, and the wasteful use of administrative resources on duplicated activity. They correctly leave to politicians the consideration of the level of central NHS funding and concentrate on ensuring that all those involved in local health care provision work together to make the best use of available resources. Their goal is to provide the most care possible to all people within a community in an equitable manner that is sensitive to their particular needs and is of the highest possible quality.

If the reforms can facilitate the achievement of that goal they will indeed have been successful. However it remains too early to assess their effect, for the simplistic counting of numbers generated by inadequate information systems does little to inform the debate (Kellner 1993), and more meaningful measures need to be established as a matter of urgency.

References

Allen, D (1989) *Lay Proposals for the Development of General Practice; A review for the Royal College of General Practitioners Patient Liaison Group* Royal College of General Practitioners.

Berwick, DM, Enthoven, A and Bunker JP (1992a) 'Quality management in the NHS: the doctor's role – I' *British Medical Journal* **304**, 235–9.

Berwick, DM, Enthoven, A and Bunker JP (1992b) 'Quality management in the NHS: the doctor's role – II' *British Medical Journal* **304**, 304–8.

BMJ (1965) 'Towards a new contract' *British Medical Journal* **5434**, 535–536.

Buck, C, Fry, J and Irvine D (1974) A framework for good primary care: The measurement and achievement of quality *Journal of the Royal College of General Practitioners* **24**, 599–604.

Buckley, EG (1989) 'Quality assessment or quality control' *Journal of the Royal College of General Practitioners* **39**, 309–312.

Cartwright and Anderson (1979) *Patients and their Doctors 1977; Report for the Royal Commission on the National Health Service* Occasional Paper 8, HMSO.

Colin-Thome, D (1992) in Pirie, A and Kelly, M. (eds) *Fund Holding: A Practice Guide* Radcliffe Medical Press, 129–131.

DoH (1988) *Promoting Better Health* Cmd No. 249, HMSO.

DoH (1989a) *General Practice in the National Health Service: A new contract* Health Departments of Great Britain.

DoH (1989b) *Practice budgets for General Medical Practitioners* Working Paper 3, NHS Review, HMSO, London.

DoH (1991) *The Patient's Charter* HMSO, London.

Eimerl, TS (1960) 'Organised curiosity' *Journal of The Royal College of General Practitioners* **3**, 246–252.

Enthoven, AC (1985) *Reflections on the Management of the National Health Service* Occasional Paper 5, Nuffield Provincial Hospitals Trust.

Essex Family Health (1992) *Quality in General Practice: The Goals for 1995* Essex Family Health.

European Conference on the teaching of general practice (1974) *The general practitioner in Europe: a statement by a Working Party of The Second European Conference on the teaching of general practice in Europe* Leewenhurst, Netherlands.

Fowler, N (1991) *Ministers Decide: A Memoir of The Thatcher Years* Chapmans, 183–198.

GMSC (1993) *The New Health Promotion Package* General Medical Services Committee, British Medical Association, February 1993.

Ham, C (1992) *Locality Purchasing* Discussion Paper 30, Health Services Management Centre, University of Birmingham.

Ham, C (1993) 'How go the NHS reforms?' *British Medical Journal* **306**, 77–78.

HSM (1991) *Not R&D but D&A* Editorial, Health Service Management, December, 1991.

Irvine, D (1983) 'Quality: our outstanding problem' *Journal of the Royal College of General Practitioners* **33**, 521–523.

Irvine, D (1990) *Managing for Quality in general practice* Medical Audit Series, King's Fund Centre.

Kellner, P (1993) 'Terminal case of truth haunts NHS' *Sunday Times* 31 January.

Lomas, J (1990) 'Quality assurance and effectiveness in healthcare: an overview,' *Quality Assurance in Health Care* **2**, 1, 5–12.

McGuiness, BW (1980) 'Why not a practice annual report?' *Journal of The Royal College of General Practitioners* **30**, 744.

Merrison, Sir A (1979) *Royal Commission on the NHS* Cmnd 7615 HMSO, London.

Morley, V (1993) 'Empowering GPs as purchasers' *British Medical Journal* **306**, 112–14.

NHSME (1992) *Local Voices: The Views of Local People in Purchasing for Health* NHS Management Executive, January 1992.

NHA (1992) *The Northampton Options in Purchasing Project. Interim and Final Reports*. Northampton Health Authority.

NHA (1993) *The Northampton Specialty Liaison Group Project* Interim Report, Northampton Health Authority.

Richards, C (1988) 'A car with flat batteries' *Journal of the Royal College of General Practitioners* **38**, 535–538.

RCGP (1985a) *Quality in General Practice* Policy Statement 2, The Royal College of General Practitioners.

RCGP (1985b) *What Sort of Doctor? Assessing Quality of Care in General Practice* Report from General Practice 23, July 1985, Royal College of General Practitioners.

Spence, Sir James (1960) *The Purpose and Practice of Medicine* Oxford University Press.

Stockport (1992) *An Approach to Locality-based Primary Care-led Strategic Management of Health Services* Stockport Health Authority and Stockport Family Health Services Authority.

Tarnowski, J (1992) *Practice Sensitive Purchasing in Bath: DHA report on the feasibility Study*.

Tomlinson, Sir Bernard (1992) *Report of the Inquiry into London's Health Service, Medical Education and Research*, HMSO, London.

Willis, A (1984) 'The need for management training in the postgraduate education of general practitioners' *Journal of the Royal College of General Practitioners* February, 116–117.

11 Of confidence and identity: the doctor in management

Michael Tremblay

Introduction

Doctors in the UK have always been involved in the management of clinical resources and some have even been more actively involved in senior management roles in hospitals. General practitioners run small and perhaps not so small businesses if some of the fundholding practices is any indication. And doctors who retain a private practice may also be investors in their own clinical facilities including hospitals. Hospital doctors in the NHS, though, appear to have been progressively disenfranchised since most hospitals were nationalised in 1948 to the point today when there is again heightened concern that doctors are not properly represented in health care management.

This chapter considers the various factors which need to be taken into account when looking at the broader issue of doctors and management. The chapter will consider a variety of 'forces' which have an impact on doctors and on management, and thereby provide a broad framework for considering doctors in management. The chapter will be divided into the following sections, each dealing with the corresponding questions:

1 Terminology: what do we call a doctor in a management role?

2 Role change: what are the factors which are active when a doctor takes on managerial responsibilities?

3 Career structure: what are the characteristics of a doctor's career which affects their exposure to management ideas and may influence their ideas about management and their place in it?

4 Educational opportunities: what courses and other educational activities are available to help a doctor who is interested in developing as a manager?

5 Competency: what does it mean to be a good manager and is being a good manager incompatible with being a good doctor?

6 Peer relationships: how does a doctor in management relate to their colleagues who are not managers, and especially to those for whom the doctor has managerial responsibility?

7 Why bother?: what incentives/disincentives are there to encourage a doctor to pursue a management-oriented career path?

Terminology

It is important to get the terminology clear. These days we often speak of front-line management, devolved management, empowerment etc to describe the pattern of cascading managerial responsibility down the organisational hierarchy. Middle managers in these organisations are at risk as management responsibility from above is given away to those below them; these managers, in turn, are challenged to prove that they are needed. Increasingly, organisations are finding that they are not needed, at least not in abundance. And, as organisations flatten, and become less hierarchical, the diffuse sharing of managerial responsibility empowers more people with management responsibility, decoupling the role of manager with the tasks of management.

To some extent, the recent past and the anticipated future, has demonstrated a preference for new managerial roles to embrace a service component as well. For example, managers who also go out on sales calls, repair equipment, or doctors in management who maintain a case-load. While dedicated middle managers may become an endangered species, the tasks of management, such as budgeting, staffing, planning and so on become tasks undertaken by increasing numbers of people, often but not always closely associated with management.

This process can be considered as either adding management tasks to a person's job, or as rethinking the organisation so that dedicated management roles become fewer as management tasks are shared out. The former for some represents 'just more work', while the latter for others represents a fundamentally new way of configuring management in modern organisations. Happily, the latter is becoming recognised as the right approach; sadly, too many organisations engage in the former.

From a traditional doctor's perspective, managers have not always been viewed kindly, Indeed, it might be characterised with considerable hostility, if not antipathy. So why would a doctor want to become a manager, this creature which causes doctors so much grief, concern and problems (at least from the doctor's point of view).

Doctors, though, are always actively involved in management. They managed the earliest hospitals, and until advances in clinical technology and the expanding role of other health professionals made personal management impossible, doctors certainly ran hospitals. General practices, too, are small businesses, which are only now being given additional purchasing power through fundholding.

Developments, such as general management, in the UK, may be seen as disenfranchising doctors from management. In part, this is due to a management paradigm, drawn from the private sector, which it was thought better fit the health field.

It is unfortunate, though, that general management thinking was introduced at the expense of a more robust concept of management involving clinicians. Industry, for example, draws its general managers from within its own staff who have had many years of management development, through schooling and experience on the job, and possess a thorough understanding of the business. Dropping general managers into health management as though health were just another product appeared to show little insight into the complexities of management of health service organisations as distinct from other types of organisations.

We are now paying for this, to some extent; doctors, who have an informed insider understanding of clinical priorities, for example, often clash with managers who are perceived to have little appreciation of the values of the health service.

Doctors can often be perceptive in their suspicion of accountancy-driven health care when governments need to create wholesale reforms to ensure that patient services and needs are paramount – through patients' charters and elaborate contracting systems.

So who is a doctor in management? The options include:

1 a doctor who is a manager;

2 a manager who is a doctor;

3 a manager who used to be a doctor;

4 a doctor who does management.

The terminology does little justice to the complexity of management and medicine. A doctor who does management engages in an activity which others might view with some consternation: can he/she be sincere; after all, there are other people who are full-time managers who do little other than manage. What if the doctor wants to get *good* at management?

Doctors do go through rigorous selection and education to become doctors, which requires well-developed numeracy skills, judgement (such as in working with incomplete information on a patient), attributes which are looked for in managers and which often underpin competency models of management.

The ambiguity in how to describe a legitimate management role for doctors does little to foster an interest in it. This may be partly because of the poor definition of the management role in the evolving NHS itself, but also because of a perception that management is not a particularly challenging or difficult activity.

So what terms might be better. I would suggest the following:

1 physician-manager;

2 physician-executive.

Physician-managers might be seen as doctors who undertake management roles below that of physician-executives who might also be understood as clinical directors or chief executive officers. At least the hyphen serves the purpose of linking two activities to which one wants to impart some sort of equality or balance and hence legitimacy to the two together. Physician-manager is the generic term.

The identity crisis, therefore, reflects profound problems for the doctor. The following sections will reflect this section's use of terminology in considering the remaining aspects of physician-managers.

Role change

It is a general characteristic of career development of professionals such as lawyers, accountants etc that in due course management roles become career possibilities. Some people, pursuing specialist qualifications in management, such as MBA degrees, arrive at management roles sooner than others. While some professionals increase the likelihood of filling management roles by acquiring specialist qualifications such as these. Doctors need to consider themselves no different from their other professional colleagues, with the exception that the career structure of doctors makes the development of management competency less certain.

However, for a significant number of professionals, the role change which occurs as they assume greater management responsibility, and thus provide less direct service (as an accountant doing the books, or engineer building bridges) will influence how they describe themselves, and how they represent themselves to their colleagues and to the public.

For hospital doctors, who arrive at the possibility of management roles after many years in a subordinate training role, for instance, which has unacknowledged management responsibilities, this presents unique problems. The career structure of doctors, culminating in a consultant post, also confers the necessary positional responsibility to undertake formal management responsibilities such as a clinical director. However, the management responsibility will usually involve responsibility for the actions of a peer group, and may involve management purview over clinical competency and clinical autonomy.

Doctors in clinical directors roles have described their relationship with their peers as one of the most challenging aspect of clinical management. Others have indicated a concern about appearing too eager to embrace their management role for fear of alienating the necessary support of their consultant colleagues.

However, doctors do successfully undertake management responsibilities throughout their medical career; the rather late formal recognition of this at the consultant level does little to encourage development of management responsibilities among more junior doctors. The role change that doctors face in formalising their managerial activities is thus made the more difficult by the failure of their career structure to acknowledge this role change. Doctors in general practice, for example, move into management as soon as they open up their practice. The labelling of general practices as businesses, though, is anathema to some, but is properly recognised in fundholding practices.

The role change is more fully understood through considering the next section of the career structure of doctors. But to summarise, doctors, while experiencing some understandable anxiety about what to call themselves so as to maintain clinical respectability, also face the fact that to move into a physician-manager role puts them into a different relationship with their colleagues. Clearly, this role is one which creates an inequality among consultants who see themselves as a peer group.

Career structure

The career structure for doctors has very specific characteristics, which reflect the interest society has in the medical profession. The career structure also reflects the historical reactions to changes and developments in medical staffing and medical hierarchies, and may be again changing in the UK in response to influences from membership in the European Community.

Various organisations, as well, take an interest in the career of the doctor. The General Medical Council sets the standards and expectations for medical education and licensing, with the Royal Colleges taking on the responsibility for specialist credentialling. The other groups are concerned with general practitioners and still others are concerned with the post-graduate education of doctors.

Within this network of interests lies a doctor who, upon graduating from medical school, undertakes a year of work prior to registration, and then makes or follows through particular career decisions.

These decisions lead our young doctor into one of the following paths:

1 hospital medicine not leading to a consultant position;

2 specialist medicine leading to a consultant position;

3 general practice.

The general approach these three career paths involve reflects distinctions between the training grades and the non-training grades of medical staffing.

The career choices, though, are daunting. Following registration, a doctor can pursue a career in general practice or begin basic specialist training. For those opting for general practice, a course, involving work as a senior house officer will lead to independent practice as a general practitioner. Some doctors, however, may not choose the GP vocational training programme, and may enter directly into general practice.

General practitioners who want to maintain an interest in hospital medicine, can become clinical assistants. This clinical assistant position can in some cases lead to a staff grade position in a hospital. Staff grade positions are newer and subject to numerical limitations. Thus, the doctor interested in general practice, can choose a route which also provides an opportunity to take on a non-training staff grade position in a hospital.

Doctors whose interests are different, pursue first a basic specialist training programme covering a number of years. Completion of this provides the opportunity to undertake higher specialist training. There is, though, the option of filling a staff grade position and leaving the training stream.

Doctors in higher specialist training act as registrars and senior registrars, and some may similarly enter a staff grade position from there. While there are limits on staff grade positions, there may be increasing pressure to create more of these roles as a way of altering the career path with respect to training posts; this would significantly alter career advancement and might force new thinking on career development outside training.

Upon completion of higher specialist training, the doctor may become a consultant. The system is fluid in the UK since changes are proposed to alter this aspect of the career structure. Alternately he/she may fill an associate specialist position, pending future vacancies.

Controlling the number of consultant positions independently of the number of people who have completed their higher specialist training creates a cadre of qualified specialists who remain in clinically supervised roles.

It is current practice for clinical directors to be consultants, ie people who have passed through all the training grades. It does appear, therefore, that doctors in non-training career paths are unlikely to be candidates for senior management roles. This does not necessarily preclude them from physician-manager roles, but the career structure does not at present offer any mechanism for how this might be done.

For some doctors, academic medicine is another opportunity with its own hierarchy of lecturer to professor, along side that of registrar to consultant. The General Medical Council in its *Recommendations on the Training of Specialists* [1987, p. 15], state: 'Training in essentially non-clinical subjects should include components of appropriate clinical experience'.

This report, though, does not mention management training and development as a formal competency of the independent practitioner, apart from the following comments [p. 6]:

understanding and appreciation of the roles, responsibilities and skills of nurses and other health care workers.

the ability to lead, guide and coordinate the work of others.

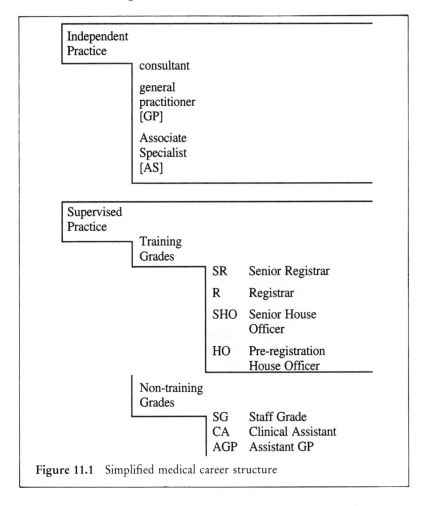

Figure 11.1 Simplified medical career structure

Acquisition of experience in administration and planning, including:

1 *efficient management of the doctor's own time and professional activities;*

2 *appropriate use of diagnostic and therapeutic resources, and appreciation of the economic and practical constraints affecting the provision of health care; and*

3 *willingness to participate, as required, in the work of bodies which advise, plan and assist the development and administration of medical services, such as NHS authorities, Royal Colleges and Faculties, and professional associations.*

Figure 11.1 represents the various career roles of doctors. It is important to add that management roles for doctors are actually undertaken throughout their career, both in and out of training. The regret is that the due recognition of these activities for career development is not readily forthcoming.

The challenge for health management is developing ways to legitimate the acquisition of appropriate management competencies along side the development of clinical competency. This would make the subsequent selection of candidates for senior management roles one of selecting from a larger and probably better prepared talent pool than is currently the case. Certainly, the doctors who aspire to or have attained management roles reflect the best management talent available; but the uncertainty of its development by doctors makes it problematic that as health service organisations seek to become better managed they will be able to find a ready source of expertise when they need it.

This last point is a general problem for health service management, ie the identification of managerial talent. Encouraging the medical profession to recognise management as a legitimate competency of some doctors would go some way to helping address the shortage of highly skilled managers which will become more acute as the reformed health service places greater and more sophisticated demands on people with management responsibilities, including doctors.

Figure 11.2 simplifies the career structure by suppressing some of the more subtle distinctions and may also not reflect the career progression of any particular doctor. This career structure in the UK is under review and may change; it is, however, broadly descriptive of the situation in March 1993.

Educational opportunities

The difficulty for doctors developing management competency is the overriding concern for clinical skill development during their training years. There are many and varied courses generally available to develop management aptitudes which would bring aspiring physician-managers into contact with others similarly disposed, but from different backgrounds.

Fitzgerald and Sturt (1992) suggest that doctors should not be developed in isolation from other types of managers. This sound advice would ensure that doctors developed appropriate understanding of how other people view their own responsibilities and problems. Doctors who have attended courses with managers from the private sector have indicated that it was helpful to share insights and learn from others new ways of looking at similar problems.

At present, there is available a wide array of courses in management in the UK, ranging from courses on the television from the Open University, to self-study management texts, to short courses to full-time post-graduate management degrees. There is, also, a tendency to look at the management development of doctors as occurring away from the

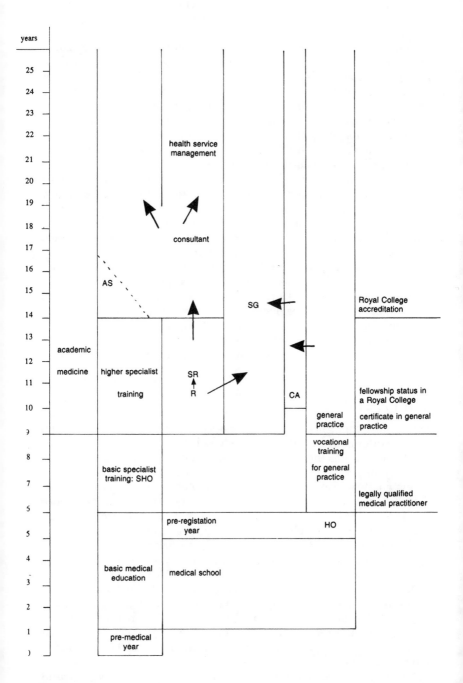

Figure 11.2　Simplified medical career structure

development of other managers. It is difficult for doctors to organise their work to attend part-time MBAs, or to undertake a short course programme.

Certainly, doctors, like anyone with an interest in learning about management, can find substantial avenues. The question is will they, and if they want to how can it be accomplished. Other methods for development of physician-managers might include formal mentoring programmes, and until there are significant numbers of respected physician-managers or physician-executives to undertake this role and act as role models, such a route must be fulfilled by non-physician-managers alone. This route offers a keen doctor the opportunity to develop appropriate management abilities.

But how can they practise what they are learning? What if they want to undertake significant clinical management responsibilities; how might this be matched against the existing career structure which puts consultants into these roles? And there is the additional issue that junior doctors rotate from place to place. Rotation through different organisational systems provides an important opportunity for the doctor to learn how other people do things, and thus bring a broad perspective to each new employer. But is anyone interested?

These questions should provide the basis for developing substantial learning opportunities for doctors interested in management, and thus go some way to addressing the need of talented physician-managers in the future. They also reflect the frustration that junior doctors feel when they go about learning about management.

Competency

Doctors are concerned with competency, managers to them appear not to be working with structured models. Doctors and managers must be developed together. It is not uncommon to hear doctors speak critically of managers. From the doctors' perspective, managers seem to get in their way, and be concerned only with financial matters. When managers speak, they use ordinary language in special and coded ways. For many people, including doctors, this 'management speak' often sounds like it ought to mean something but a lack of familiarity with management models can make access to the meanings difficult.

It is in fact the use of management models that might be surprising to many non-managers. Indeed, the past 100 years has seen the development of many models of management, from Frederick Taylor's scientific management through various schools of thinking to today's ideas. Today, many of these models and ideas of management may appear to some to lack scientific rigour, to be a product of a popular management culture, an issue of management fashion and trend and not rational thought.

Much of management thinking, though, does rest on simple truths about how to treat a fellow human being, about basic notions of ethical conduct, as well as researched work on human motivation and behaviour, financial controls and information technology.

For doctors who have undertaken a fundamentally scientific programme of study, and who work with data, dealing with the softer issues of human relationships in the workplace and motivation challenges their own well-developed methods of analysis.

Certainly, there is no reason why a doctor should not be able to comprehend financial accounting, statistical and other data. Working with data is part of their own medical education. Similarly, doctors should be able to use this information to inform decision-making and planning about allocation of health resources.

The important difference for a doctor and a manager is that while the doctor is concerned about this or that particular patient, managers are concerned with types or groups of patients. A doctor faced with dealing with a patient for whom a recommended procedure is unavailable has a human problem of their relationship to each patient; a manager faced with the same problem, is dealing with rationing, and the efficacy of the intervention in patients of similar type.

For the physician-manager it is necessary to balance these potentially conflicting perspectives. Being good, then, as a physician and a manager may emerge from the turmoil of the issues as much as from being able to exhibit technical competence in a variety of tasks, for example.

There are many models of competency: from the Management Charter Initiative dealing with general managerial competence, to specific competencies associated with open learning courses, to standards such as are found in managerial accreditation systems in Canada and the United States.

The challenge for doctors and managers in the UK is developing a model of managerial competency that works for health service management, reflecting its unique characteristics. For doctors interested in management, they should exercise critical caution and ensure that the management skills, and abilities they learn are appropriate to the nature of their management responsibilities, and are based on acceptable ethical and value considerations.

Peer relationships

This chapter has referred to the importance of the peer relationship to doctors. For doctors in management, maintaining working clinical relationships with colleagues is imperative. However, a management role is *primus inter pares* – it makes the physician-manager first among equals.

For example, the physician-manager faces significant managerial responsibilities which could imbalance the peer relationships:

1 the management of resources such as money, support personnel, clinical equipment;

2 the management of terms and conditions of employment including increasingly being involved in hiring new consultants or being involved in decision-making about who is hired, and the contractual expectations of the position;

3 the responsibility for ensuring that the other staff, including the medical staff, are carrying out their responsibilities which may involve simply ensuring that the clinical services are provided, but may involve formal review of clinical performance and a veto role over the use of junior medical staff or others by consultant colleagues.

Wanting to maintain a balanced clinical relationship with colleagues may not always be compatible with the expectations of the managerial role. More participative and democratic management styles, compatible with collegial working relationships, may give way to authoritarian or high-handed decision-making when there are problems which cannot be resolved to everyone's satisfaction. The former will please the physician-manager's colleagues, the latter foster ill-will. The latter style may also bring charges that the physician-manager has been coopted by management, has 'gone over to the other side', and thus further attenuate the goodwill.

Managing professionals, such as doctors by other doctors, will always face these complications. This is no reason, however, to avoid the responsibility.

Why bother?

Of course, thinking about doctors in management asks the question 'why bother?' Why bother encouraging doctors to become involved in management. Is it not sufficient that doctors play a significant role in the health of people and the resources to help them, is it not sufficient that it does not make much sense to suggest that doctors needed a particular rationale for wanting to become involved in management, is it not sufficient that organisations should want to identify all their talented people for management, and not make certain assumptions about fitness to be a manager. After all, such assumptions often have the effect of discriminating against talented people for failing to have certain characteristics and not others.

There is the argument from self-defence: if doctors do not fill appropriate management roles, others will and they may deal with the important issues in ways that doctors feel are inappropriate. Of course, the challenge to the physician-manager in this case is that the management responsibilities do not empower them to acquiesce to their colleagues' desires. The physician-manager is now responsible for other health professionals, support staff, and all their requirements and expectations.

There is the argument from ability: doctors are capable of learning the requisite skills of management, and being very good at them. This challenge adds to the doctor's repertoire of talent and may arguably be a good thing in itself. There is also the argument from added value: a doctor brings to the management role an important perspective that has often been absent around the management table. By being involved as a physician-manager, the doctor ensures that the management processes reflect a broader consensus of opinion. Importantly, too, the doctor is a key determinant in how clinical resources are allocated and utilised; the physician-manager is thereby able to integrate clinical accountability for effective resource use with the management of resource use.

Conclusions
The way forward

This chapter has addressed a variety of factors, which describe the doctor in management. The following conclusions are also calls to action by doctors and managers and by physician-managers, to better define the management role of doctors, and to ensure that talented doctors pursue appropriate management careers with full recognition and support of their physician colleagues.

Terminology

While what we call things is often arbitrary, it is important to develop language with which we can become comfortable, and which conveys meanings that can be shared by all. Legitimating specific terminology for doctors in management roles, such as physician-managers moves toward words which can embody meanings which other doctors can accept, and which other managers can understand. The effect will be to empower the doctor as a manager, with the respect of her colleagues or other managers.

Role change

It would seem appropriate to consider what can be done to support doctors as they become physician-managers, with particular concern for ensuring that they move into this role with the full support of their colleagues, including other consultants.

Career structure

The identification of management talent among doctors is complicated by the almost exclusive focus on clinical development during the training of doctors. Recent trends to expect consultants to have done some management training serves to trivialise the importance of developing the role of physician-manager. Doctors do do management throughout their training and it must be acknowledged and made explicit. Career development for those who seek enhanced management roles should incorporate appropriate expectations of ability. Importantly, though, the career structure needs to make the management role more pervasive throughout, and not something that can be formally identified only at the consultant level.

Educational opportunities

Doctors will need to be able to practise their budding management talents. We need to know how they can do this and have it recognised as an important part of their own professional clinical development. This is not for all doctors, but it is for those who will fill the physician-manager roles of the future.

Competency

It is probably timely for the UK to consider establishing appropriate management accreditation for senior health service managers. The responsibilities of management today are more complex and demanding than in the past and the public needs assurance that its health institutions are in capable hands. Similarly, for doctors interested in management careers, recognition of the legitimate competencies associated with the physician-manager role would enhance their credibility and warrant increased peer support.

Why bother?

Recognition of a proper role for the physician-manager is timely and appropriate. The effective use of scarce resources in health has heightened society's awareness of the difficulties faced in responding to apparent limitless demand for health care. Physician-managers can bridge this gulf between public understanding and the setting of health service priorities. It is time for the medical profession to recognise this important role and to ensure that interested doctors can pursue meaningful and acknowledged career paths leading to leadership roles in management.

Statistics on doctors

Table 11.1 Numbers of doctors in non-training positions, by sex

	Total	Male	Female	Year
AGP	425	174	251	1 October 1991
		41%	59%	
AS	844	523	321	30 September 1990
		62%	38%	
CA	7714	5379	2335	30 September 1990
		70%	30%	
SG	488	342	146	30 September 1991
		70%	30%	

Source: SCOPME April 1992

Table 11.2 Average age of staff grade [SG] doctors

	Average age	Average male age	Average female age
SG	41	28.64	28.59

Source: SCOPME April 1992

Table 11.3 Career movement into the staff grade

Into SG	from	Number	Percentage
	R	175	37.9
	CA	129	27.9
	Locum	66	14.3
	SHO	51	11.0
	Other	31	6.7
	SR	10	2.2
	total	462	100.0

Source: SCOPME April 1992

Table 11.4   Numbers of doctors by career step

Position	Number	Total	Percentage
Consultant		13672	35.1
Other		2932	7.6
Staff grade, Associate Specialist,			
Hospital GPs etc	488		
Junior grades		22305	57.3
Senior registrar	2980		
Registrar	5823		
Senior house officer	10563		
House officer	2939		
Total		38909	100.0

Source: SCOPME April 1992

References

Curry, L (1989) 'Identification of functionally necessary knowledge and skills in the practice of Canadian health care management' *Journal of Health Education Administration* **7**, 47–69

Ellis, R (ed.) (1988) *Professional Competence and Quality Assurance in the Caring Professions* Chapman and Hall

Fitzgerald, L and Sturt J (1992) 'Clinicians into management: on the change agenda or not? *Health Services Management Research* **5**, 137–146

General Medical Council (1987) *Recommendations on the Training of Specialists* October 1987

Harrison, S, Hunter, DJ, Marnock, G and Pollitt, C (1989) 'General management and medical autonomy in the National Health Service' *Health Service Management Research* **2**, 38–46

Johnson, JA and Boss, RW (1991) 'Management development and change in a demanding health care environment' *Journal of Management Development* **10**, 5–10

KET Foundation Inc. (1984) *The Business of Managing Professionals*

Pollitt, C *et al.* (1988) 'The reluctant managers: clinicians and budgets in the NHS' *Financial Accountability and Management* **4**, 213–233

SCOPME (1992) *Working Paper on the Educational Needs of the Staff Grade and Other Groups* London, April 1992

Sternberg, RJ and Killigian, J (1990) *Competence Considered* Yale University Press

Stewart, R and Dopson S (1988) 'Griffiths in theory and practice: a research assessment' *Journal of Health Administration Education* **6**, 503–514

Tremblay, M (1993) *Evaluation Report of Clinicians in the Senior Executive Course at Manchester Business School* HSMC, March 1993

Tremblay, M (in the press) *Senior Registrar Management Development* HSMC

Willis, SL and Dubin, SS (eds) (1990) *Maintaining Professional Competence* Jossey-Bass

12 Community care

Anne Davis

Introduction

The Government's Community Care reforms described in this chapter were envisaged to be fully implemented from April 1991. However, the Secretary of State, Kenneth Clarke, announced in July 1991 that the reforms would be phased in over three financial years, with the transfer of funding from DSS to local authorities not taking place till April 1993. Thus, some of the areas covered by this revised chapter have been progressed, whilst others, in particular the assessment and financial aspects of community care are only now being implemented.

The stated objective of central government policy towards community care is summarised in the White Paper *Caring for People* as: (DHSS 1989a)

> *to enable people to live as normal a life as possible, with the right amount of care and support to achieve maximum possible independence, while giving people a greater individual say in how they live their lives and the services they need to help them to do so.*

This enabling approach to community care is shared by the majority of managers and professional people who plan and deliver health and social services, and is the foundation upon which many examples of existing good practice have been built. The implementation of the new proposals are the responsibility of Local Authorities and alter the relationships, not only between social services and District Health Authorities, but also between the public and private sectors. However, their success or failure will be measured by the people who receive the service – the users and their carers. This chapter will consider the principles, objectives and key changes contained in *Caring for People* from the consumer perspective, and assess whether the proposals seem likely to achieve the Government's stated intention, given the changing interface between the public and private sectors.

The challenge for health and social services

Providing adequate levels of care to meet the needs of the rapidly increasing numbers of elderly and very elderly people is the biggest challenge facing health and social services in the 1990s. However, community care means more than this, and, according to the government's definition, it includes:

providing the services and support which people who are affected by problems of ageing, mental illness, mental handicap or physical or sensory disability need to be able to live as independently as possible in their own homes, or in 'homely' settings in the community . . . which enables such people to achieve their full potential.

Local Authority social services departments are responsible for the provision of community services. They take the lead, in collaboration with medical, nursing and other interests, in assessing individual need, designing care arrangements and securing their delivery within available resources. Social services departments have become the budget-holders for a range of community care services, including financial support of people in private and voluntary homes. However, they are no longer to be the main providers of community services, and will be closely monitored to ensure they plan and provide services in line with central government policy. Social services will carry substantial responsibilities, but will have limited power and cash-limited resources. NHS community service delivery has not transferred to Local Authorities, but must be jointly planned with social services.

The Government's plans to reform the structure and management of community care will have far-reaching implications for managers and users of both health and social services. The policy of transferring responsibility for continuing care from the NHS to local authorities, together with a renewed emphasis on the private/voluntary sector as providers of residential care are explicit, but the private and voluntary sectors are also to be offered 'ample scope' to provide community health and social services to people living in their own home. There are no proposals for monitoring this aspect of community care.

New arrangements for joint planning of services and the financing of community care are intended to alter the relationship between the National Health Service, local government and the independent sector. Indeed, the success or failure of the reforms may well depend on the ability of these professionals to collaborate effectively in multi-disciplinary and multi-sector teams.

Government policy objectives

It is clear that the philosophy underlying the community care reforms is consistent with other changes introduced by central government during the 1980s, both for the National Health Services and local government. To place it in its proper setting, the National Health Service and Community Care Act (1989), which enacts the proposals contained in *Working for Patients* (DHSS 1989b) and *Caring for People* (DHSS 1989a) must be measured against *Promoting Better Health* (DHSS, 1987), the Local Government and Housing Act (HMSO 1989a) and the Education Act (HMSO 1989b). These pieces of legislation exemplify central government commitment to devolve power towards the consumers or users of the services, to cash limit public spending, to separate the providers and the purchasers of services, to introduce market forces and to encourage a mixed economy – the emphasis on private rather than public sector provision.

Caring for People explicitly states that its focus is on clarifying roles and responsibilities, to establish an effective financial and managerial framework for service delivery in line with national policy objectives. It does not, however, define the differences between 'social care' and 'health care' which has been a central point of confusion for managers monitoring the private sector, where clear distinctions are demanded by the legal differences between residential homes and nursing homes.

As in other areas of policy, the Government has encouraged the expansion of private health and social care since 1979, and there has been a massive 'silent revolution' as one of the biggest privatisation programmes progressed with surprisingly little public debate. It is ironic that growing concern about the rapidly increasing cost of supporting people, particularly elderly people, in *private* residential and nursing homes, has prompted the Government's intervention in community care.

The social security budget of £10 million in 1980 multiplied a hundred-fold to £1 billion in 1989 and is now estimated to be £2500 million. This massive increase occurred as the private sector responded to the demand for residential care, while the public sector provision of domiciliary health and social services failed to keep pace with increasing numbers of elderly people. The Audit Commission (1986) reported in 1986 that, by providing open-ended public funding for people in residential and nursing homes, while restricting the support available to people living in their own homes, the Government had created a 'perverse incentive' for people to enter expensive residential care.

Following this report, the Minister of Health invited Sir Roy Griffiths to make recommendations about the structure and management of community care, but his recommendations were to be on a nil cost basis. The contrast between the enthusiastic reception given to the long-awaited Griffiths Report, '*Community Care – An Agenda for Action* (Griffiths 1988), and the considerable scepticism with which the Government's response was greeted, was strongest on two fundamental issues: central government's reluctance to place community care more firmly under social services control, as recommended by the Griffiths Report, and the appropriate method of funding.

Funding community care

The Minister of Health's initial refusal to make a specific 'ring-fenced' grant to finance the rapidly growing budget for care in the community led Sir Roy Griffiths to declare his disappointment that, whereas he had designed 'a purposeful, effective four-wheel vehicle', the White Paper had redesigned it as a three-wheeler. There was widespread anxiety that, unless there is ring-fencing, the central government money which is transferred from social security to social services budgets, may be diverted to other Local Authority services. These fears were expressed by organisations invited to give evidence to the Social Services Select Committee of the House of Commons. The third report of the Committee recommended that the Department of Health look again at the ring-fencing of social services budgets, but also at NHS community funding 'in the light of fears that Health Authorities' budgets could be raided by the acute sector' (House of Commons Social Services Committee 1990). When the funding of community care was eventually announced in October 1992, there was a last minute change-of-heart and the Secretary of State, Virginia Bottomley, included 'special levers and controls': ie the ring-fencing of the Special Transitional Grant money, this included the direction that 85 per cent of the money allocated for care in the community must be used to fund care provided by the independent sector.

However, there was a deeper worry, beyond the issue of ring-fencing, that the funds would simply be insufficient to bridge the gap (estimated in 1990 to be £30 to £40 per week) which already existed between the fees for residential and nursing home care and the social security payments to meet these costs. During the debate on the Second Reading of the Health Service and Community Care Bill on March 15 1990 (Hansard 1990), MPs gave many examples of the awful effects of this shortfall in funding on the lives of frail, elderly people living in private and voluntary homes who face possible eviction. The surprise Government defeat on the principle of income support for people in residential care, which followed the debate, illustrates the Government's dilemma in funding care for people living in residential settings. An extra increase in allowances was announced as a quick response from the Social Security Minister, but the underlying problems remain.

The Government announced a delay of two years in the implementation of the reforms in the summer of 1990 because of the difficulty in reaching agreement on the method of calculating the resources to be transferred to Local Authorities. Representatives of interested Government departments and Local Authority associations (the 'Algebra Group') tried to reach agreement between August 1991 and May 1992, but failed to produce an acceptable formula for transfer. The calculation was complex as it included estimating the income support that would be payable under the present system, the normal income support and housing benefit (now residential allowance) that will be payable to new residents, the continuing commitment to those residents with preserved rights under the current scheme, and the rate at which local authorities will assume responsibility for the care of new clients.

When the Secretary of State announced the global figures (£399 million to be transferred in 1993/94) and the method of its distribution in October 1992, there was an outcry at an estimated shortfall of £289 million. A technical error led to a further revision of the figures and Local Authorities had only four months to prepare to implement the changes. Local Authorities, voluntary groups and private agencies shared a common concern that the funding would be insufficient, and although revised figures reduced the estimated gap to £135 million, this is unevenly distributed and limits the services available in some Authorities.

These concerns were echoed by the House of Commons Health Committee's Third Report (1993) *Community Care: Funding from April 1993*, which concluded that 'the new funding arrangements, and the formula for calculating DSS transfer in particular, are devised in such a way as to allow little flexibility in the system should the calculations prove to be incorrect'.

Collaboration between Local Authorities and the NHS was seen to be of such central importance to successful implementation of the new community care arrangements that the Government made the payment of the grant conditional on them having provided evidence of agreement in key areas: jointly agreed strategies for placing people in nursing homes, the likely numbers involved during 1993/94, and how hospital discharge arrangements would be integrated with assessment arrangements for providing care between Health and Local Authorities (Foster-Laming letter: Chief Social Services Inspector and Deputy Chief Executive of the NHS Management Executive 25 September 1992 to Directors of Social Services and Health Authority General Managers).

In 1990 there were more than a quarter of a million places provided in residential and nursing homes, with at least 176,000 people claiming some level of benefit. Official statistics indicate that in 1991 there were 289,900 places in residential care homes (97,900 Local Authority; 36,700 voluntary; 155,300 private) and 109,000 places in nursing homes. (Health Committee 1993). There will be a perpetual struggle for higher levels of payment to meet ever-increasing fees, and a powerful lobby of organised home owners and families, with relatives in residential care, will continue to argue for more and more of the available funding to support the particularly disadvantaged people in community- based institutional care, leaving community care under-resourced.

Continuing care for elderly people, people with mental illness and people with learning difficulty has long been the Cinderella service. It is now the centre of attention and has, through social security payments, received huge amounts of extra public funding directed towards the care of some of the most socially disadvantaged people. Will the demographic changes which provide a large, articulate and active elderly population for the first time in Britain (a third of the population being over 65 years) mean that demands for better quality care for elderly people will allow these services to retain the more favoured position achieved in the past ten years? Or will individuals who wish to remain in their own homes, and their carers, find themselves ill matched in any future fight for 'available' resources?

This is the challenge facing health and social services. If they fail, the present pattern in which escalating costs have merely transferred across from health to social security will continue. Community care is not a cheap option and there is no guarantee that future services to people at home will cost less than residential care. Demand can be expected to rise as people become better informed when community care plans are published. Concern about the level of demand and the legal rights of individuals to a service to meet the needs which have been assessed has caused the SSI Chief, Herbert Laming, to emphasise that authorities do not have a duty to assess on request, but only when they think that a person may be in need of a service they provide: and that the assessment of need and the decision about the services to be provided are separate stages in the process because the second stage must take account of the resources available to the authority. Thus assessment is a tool for rationing the service to fit within the resource constraints set by the Government grant. What will be needed is proper costing of the services and adequate funding to meet those costs as demand increases.

It is important to realise that the people receiving health care in their own homes or in residential care homes will continue to be entitled to the full range of NHS services, but those who enter nursing homes become private patients, entitled only to GP and dental services and NHS hospital care when required. *Caring for People* recognised that community care puts new pressures on the NHS community health services, but Health Authorities have not received a transfer of resources to meet their enhanced responsibilities. There is no evidence that Health Authorities have increased the number of community or district nurses to support more people in their own homes, indeed many are known to have cut the number of health visitors and district nurses. The increasing number of GP fundholders further complicates the pattern. They have no incentive to purchase expensive nursing home care or to purchase community nursing services and have had little involvement in the planning of community care with the Local Authorities.

Housing and community care

Since community care is really about providing services to people who live in their own home, a brief look at government housing policy is necessary. Inadequate or inappropriate housing is often a major factor contributing to demands for health and social services. The White Paper refers to recent reforms in local government and housing which have enabled Local Authorities to provide specific assistance to elderly people and their carers for minor works in their homes. Housing associations are developing purpose-designed units for older people, but, for most frail, elderly people this type of care is inaccessible. However, the relationship between housing policy and the new private residential and nursing home pattern of care is even more significant, because elderly people who own their own homes, but have low incomes, must sell their property to finance their care when they enter a residential or nursing home.

The Government has encouraged home ownership, but these homes must be sold to pay for care in old age if an elderly person enters residential or nursing home care. There is a stark contrast between the procedures for the normal sale of a purchase of a house, and the way in which many elderly people find themselves 'placed' in their new home by professionals or relatives, and must then sell their own home to pay for care.

If we consider the rights of people in residential care in terms of housing, some of the main points of concern are bought sharply into focus. For example, legal contracts, security of tenure and fair rents are taken for granted. Under the Housing Act 1989, tenants have the right to vote so that their home is not sold over their heads. None of these rights pertain for most people in residential care. Residential and nursing homes are brought and sold as 'going concerns' (with people as stock on the shelf) and the threat of eviction faces many when their money from the sale of their house runs out and they can no longer afford the fees.

The development of residential and nursing home care from private hotels for gentlefolk, or homes run by religious orders and the military is an accident of history. Although the Registered Homes Act (HMSO 1984) was consolidated in 1984, it originates from the Nursing Homes Registration Act 1927 and the National Assistance Act 1948. Many of the homes registered were built and formerly run as hotels, and that is the basis of the system, with residents consequently having few of the rights associated with housing provision. They are treated as if they were staying in a hotel, even the social security benefit is expressed as 'bed and breakfast'. This means that many characteristics of their care are directly comparable with homeless people – not so far from the days of the workhouse, and inappropriate for 'homely' care in the 1990s.

Caring at home

Action in housing will need to be an integral part of plans to provide services in line with the first of the White Paper's six key objectives for the service delivery of community care:

> *to promote the development of domiciliary, day and respite services to enable people to live in their own homes wherever feasible and sensible.*

This objective has received universal support and is fully in line with the movement towards 'normalised' or ordinary pattens of living for elderly people, people with disabilities and people with learning difficulties. This new attitude to care has made slow progress since it became government policy in the 1970s when philosophies of health care began to move away from institutional, medical models, towards a diversity of community-based schemes, and the closure of long-stay mental handicap and psychiatric hospitals. The ordinary life philosophy has been welcomed by service users and their carers, but has sometimes placed a heavy burden on families. Fewer people are now admitted to hospital for treatment and others return home who would formerly have been kept in hospital much longer.

The most effective community care is that which empowers people to be in control of their own life, independent of others. *Caring for People* recognises that, when extra care is needed, it comes to most people, not from public services, but from families and friends. Support for the carers is the second key objective:

> *to ensure that service providers make practical support for carers a high priority.*

In their response to the White Paper, The Equal Opportunities Commission (1990) states that, 'unlike child-rearing, caring for the elderly and disabled is an open-ended task which grows more onerous over the years bringing cumulative disadvantage which may ultimately result in an impoverished old age for the carer', and they express grave reservations about the assumptions made about the increasing involvement of families in community care. The Commission points out that 'family care' may be a euphemism for 'care by the nearest female relative' and warns that the Government can no longer assume that women will continue to bear the immediate and long-term costs of community care policies.

The estimated 6 million carers are a main plank in the Government's new structure for care in the community, but little concrete evidence has yet emerged of plans to offer support to carers. At present one third of carers get no professional help at all. Their desperate need for help is illustrated in the 1992 report from the Carers National Association *Speak Up. Speak Out*, which reveals that of every three people who look after a sick, disabled or elderly relative, two become ill as a result. Half of carers are in financial difficulties and state benefits are inadequate. Two thirds of carers are over 55 years old, but invalid care allowance is not paid to retired people, therefore only 2 per cent of carers receive benefit. The financial, health and emotional problems are not transitory, over a third of the respondents in the survey had been caring for more than ten years. There are other anomalies in these assumptions about carers, not least, the changing patterns of employment as women are encouraged to stay in the labour force. The trend towards the old looking after the very old, is not a happy retirement prospect for men or women with elderly relatives and friends.

The existing government fund to support highly dependent people with the most severe disabilities, the Independent Living Fund, closed on 25 November and has been transferred to a successor trust. The Local Authority will be expected to make a contribution by way of a services equivalent to what would have been spent on residential or nursing care and the fund will provide cash payments in addition where necessary. Funding of adaptations to people's homes has been transferred to Local Authority Housing Departments who must provide disabled facility grants to enable people to remain in their own home. This change, although welcome in principle, has caused great anxiety to carers.

Assessment of individual need

Caring for People states that promoting choice underlies the Government's proposals, but determines that, in future, it will be the responsibility of Social Services Authorities to ensure that multi-disciplinary assessments are made where necessary to enable them to discharge their responsibilities. The White Paper states:

> the cornerstone of good quality care will be the proper assessment of need and good case management.

Assessment of need as perceived by professionals, and individuals and carers may appear to some as a contradiction in terms. However, it is fair to say that there is agreement amongst the public and professionals alike, that the present system of allowing self-referral, followed by automatic public financial support (regardless of the need for residential care), does not provide either good value for the taxpayer or appropriate care for many residents.

Lady Wagner, in her report *Residential Care: A Positive Choice* (Wagner 1988), highlighted the importance for service users of making real choices about the kind of care to best meet their own needs. The intention of the Secretary of State for Health is that from April 1993 Local Authorities will be responsible, in collaboration with health care professionals, for assessing the needs of new applicants for public support for residential or nursing home care and that:

> a nursing home place should only be secured if the assessment establishes a need for nursing care as the whole or main component of care required.

Clarification will be needed about the ability of residential homes to admit a person who requires nursing care, even if it is not the main component of care required. As the law stands, residential homes cannot legally accept a person who needs nursing care. Similarly, the final decision about 'nursing cases' under the new arrangements for assessment is confusing when the provisions of the NHS and Community Care Act are compared with the Registered Homes Act. A particular question is whether registration officers will retain their powers not only to register and inspect nursing homes, but also to have the final say about 'nursing', as set out in the guidance to Local Authorities under the 1984 Act.

Care managers will also be expected to be client advocates. This conflicts with their role of assessors or 'gatekeepers', since assessment of need is to be the determining factor of access to public funding for those who cannot afford to purchase appropriate services – whether provided by public, private or voluntary agencies. Their role will be similar to that held by general practitioners who become budget-holders under the new arrangements, and similar reservations have been expressed about patient choice when GPs contract for services.

The White Paper stated high ideals:

> *The objective of assessment is to determine the best possible way to help the individual ... assessments should take account of the wishes of the individual and his or her carer, and of the carer's ability to continue to provide care, and where possible should include their active participation. Efforts should be made to offer flexible services which enable individuals and carers to make choices.*

The requirements to have a common process for assessment for a range of services and to 'establish and make public criteria of eligibility for assessment, and the way in which their assessment processes will work' are welcome, but unhappily, these good intentions are undermined by the recommended action which follows assessment. Decisions on service provision will have to take account of what is available and affordable. Even if a person is assessed as needing residential care, and wishes to take that option, it may no longer be available:

> *The Government believes that, subject to the availability of resources, people should be able to exercise the maximum possible choice about the home they enter.*

It is evident that the choices of the individual patient and their carers will be restricted by the new system, as William Liang (Liang and Buisson 1989) suggests, the contracts agreed between social services and the independent providers of care will result in choices being restricted because social services are likely to be limited by cost constraints to contracting with homes at the cheaper end of the market in any district. Acknowledging the failure of the new system to provide greater choice, the Secretary of State issued a directive to ensure that when residential care is the preferred care option, people must be offered at least a choice between two establishments by the Local Authority.

However well-intentioned assessors may be, in reality, the community care proposals, designed to take us into the twenty-first century, will bear a remarkable resemblance to the poor law days of the nineteenth century – can assessors avoid making the distinction between the 'deserving' poor who match the stated objectives, priorities and budgets, and the 'undeserving' poor who do not? And will the budget-holders or managers of long-stay and acute hospital beds exert pressure so that the assessors become the consumers of the service, purchasing inappropriate care because it is too slow or too expensive to provide the package the user really wants?

As the Act stands, the public will be told the rules of the game, but they will have no right of appeal against the decision of the referee. A complaints procedure is promised, but a system of appeal is essential, particularly as the wishes of the person assessed and their carers may be in conflict. Therefore complaints and appeals procedures must also extend to carers.

We can be optimistic that this view will be shared by senior professionals. Graham Gatehouse, Director of Social Services in Surrey, has suggested some key points (Gatehouse 1990) which must underpin every successful individual care programme. He says that a care programme should:

- resolve or relieve the basic problem in a way recognised by the client as helpful;

- offer involvement of the client in the care plan process and provide an element of choice within the pan;

- be cost-effective with specification based on known costs;

- be objective and the content of plan recorded and monitored;

- have one person responsible for progressing the plan and its review;

- support the client in their own home or aid a return home;

- positively consider and act upon support for carers;

- make available complaints and appeals procedures.

The problem for potential users of the new services will be to know how to gain access into the system. *Caring for People* asserts that no one assessed as needing residential care should be deprived of the opportunity to enter an independently run home meeting the required standard of care. This begs the question of the problems facing care managers with a cash-limited budget which may run dry before the end of the year. It is also simplistic, in that it does not recognise the important differences outlined above, between residential and nursing care.

Another danger is that, because of pressures on staff, multi-disciplinary assessment may only be available to those who seek the more expensive types of care. Residential care might then become the first option, not the least, as it would open gateways to more services. On the other hand, if residential care is always the last option, could it not become stigmatised once again?

Some people 'need' residential care on different terms; they choose it because they feel safer, less lonely, and enjoy being looked after for the first time in their lives! In future, this real choice will only be open to people who can afford to pay for themselves. There can be little doubt that the Government's proposals will widen the gap between publicly funded and private patients, a difference that good home owners presently seek to minimise.

Implications for NHS acute services

The implications of community care arrangement are pertinent to managers of acute and long-stay wards for elderly patients in the NHS. Many elderly people will return to the community after multidisciplinary assessment in hospital but there has been widespread concern that some patients are put into homes when doctors face pressures to use beds 'blocked' by frail elderly patients.

District Health Authorities are developing plans, in line with Government policy, to replace most of the continuing care beds in geriatric wards with beds provided by voluntary nursing homes. In this case, the new discharge procedure (DoH 1989a) is applicable. The guidance from the Department of Health prohibits the discharge of a patient to a nursing or residential home in which they must pay for their care, without their consent. This consent must extend to the family of the patient who will also be affected by any transfer from free NHS care into the private sector.

This policy of reducing the number of geriatric beds holds another inherent danger for the NHS, particularly for those districts which have closed all their long-stay provision. Managers will want to consider the transient nature of many of the existing nursing homes, with rapid changes of ownership and much financial instability. The private sector has expanded rapidly under favourable financial circumstances. There is no guarantee that all existing nursing homes will continue in business when assessment and contracts for service under the new financial arrangements are introduced, and some homes will be closed down by inspectors because of low standards. Acute beds could then be the only fall-back for people in need of nursing care and with nowhere else to go. For example, an emergency closure of a nursing home in Harrogate on New Year's Eve, 1988, caused the Health Authority to re-open a hospital ward to accommodate the patients in safety.

It has been estimated that there may presently be a 30 per cent over-provision of places. Since the purpose of assessment is to reduce the admissions to residential care, the independent sector is becoming increasingly nervous of the short-term and longer-term future of their industry. The down-turn in the economy, including plummeting property values, has already seen many homes become bankrupt and go into liquidation. Any slowing up of admissions or reduction in overall numbers will impact quickly, particularly in areas with large numbers of vacancies already, for example the south and west of England. Occupancy levels are crucial to the profitability and survival of each business. To overcome the problems associated with assessment which may reduce their clients, some homes are applying for dual registration (as both residential care and nursing homes) while a few others are developing day care or home care services. This is changing the nature of existing homes and is not always compatible with the principles of care, which assume that these institutions are a person's own 'home'.

Community care plans must take this into full account. The boom in residential and nursing homes during the 1980s was a response to the financial gains to be made through investment in these businesses which coincided with a rapidly increasing market because of demographic change. But the majority of private homes would not have opened to admit the large numbers of people needing care unless public funds had been available. If public funding is restricted, the 'industry' could collapse, with catastrophic effect for the NHS which still has an obligation to provide services. The introduction of Hospital Trusts and general practitioners' new contracts put further pressure on the proposed structures for community care.

Community care plans

The second major change identified in *Caring for People* is that Local Authorities will be expected to produce and publish clear plans for the development of community care services, consistent with the plans of Health Authorities and other interested agencies.

Joint planning was introduced in the 1970s in the early days of the movement from long-stay hospital care to community developments for people with learning difficulties and mental illness. Its limited success is noted in the White Paper, which proposes a much more formal approach for inter-authority collaboration. It is a system which gives to central government the power of veto.

> The Government will take new powers to ensure that plans are open to inspection, and to call for reports from social services authorities.

Collaborative working is to be set in the 'new world' of a mixed economy of care, a world in which there is a clear distinction between purchasers and providers of health or social care. Local accountability is to be increased as objective setting and monitoring shift towards 'outcomes' and away from the 'machinery' or process. The Government believes that health and social services managers will see that it is in everyone's best interest to collaborate, and that the need to achieve value for public money will encourage 'both sides' to plan and work more closely. It remains to be seen if it is possible to achieve this when divisions are built into the system proposed, and many existing conflicts of interest remain. For example, there may be differences between the standards set and enforced for nursing homes and those for residential homes. Difficulties with dual registration have shown the potential for conflict, with the homes and their residents confused and uncertain about their future as health and social services disagree on standards and procedures.

On the other hand, many aspects of these proposals can be welcomed wholeheartedly. They present a challenge which seems to be enthusiastically taken up by many Health and Local Authorities in the heady atmosphere of the modern consumerism. Everyone agrees that the public need to be informed about the services available, and told how they can get help when they need it. Very real questions are raised about who is the real consumer, and how the plans will meet the express needs of users. As has been pointed out, care managers will have enormous power and will become the consumers, making decisions about the services to be purchased for users. There is provision that users of services may be consulted, but little evidence that users have been involved in drawing up the plans.

The plans outline what exists, they may indicate what the Local Authority can afford to do, it is not clear that they will try to find out from people what level of care and support is really needed and involve users in planning in an innovative way. The rhetoric of the White Paper is about involving and enabling users, but, in reality, services are to be developed for people who must submit to a professional assessment to see which service they fit into, rather than developing packages of services according to individual need. It has been suggested that *Caring for People* is a 'massive exercise in damage limitation', rather than a brave new world with a vision of enabling disadvantaged people to enjoy the benefits of community life which services have in the past so often failed to provide. The issue of identifying 'unmet needs' has taken centre stage in 1993 as the Government has become nervous of the way assessment may identify needs which resources cannot satisfy. Indeed, Government guidance from the Cabinet Office, relating to the rights embodied in the Citizens Charter, has suggested that Local Authorities must be careful to avoid individuals bringing legal action against them by planning care packages which relate to what is available rather than what is needed. In effect, this means ensuring that clients are not informed in writing of the needs which have been identified but which cannot be met. This has been described by Local Authority Associations as an invitation to assessors 'to be economical with the truth'. The House of Commons Health Committee highlighted their own concerns, stating that current Government guidance is 'unhelpful' and recommending that, if necessary, legislation be introduced 'to make sure that there are no inhibitions on the ability of Social Services Departments and Health Authorities to make a full assessment of unmet needs'.

Provision for the private sector to be involved in planning services is proposed. But who is 'the private sector'? Since private community care providers are often small businesses in competition with each other, some difficulties may be anticipated. Owner associations are suggested as the link, but how representative are they of the views of home owners? Some of the most 'homely' community care is provided by small, independent owners who are likely to be squeezed out by larger charities and international companies who will move in and bid keenly, offering economies of scale, rather than the traditional pattern of smaller homes. Some concern has already been expressed about the concentration of ownership of acute private hospitals, and registration officers report that larger homes are now being built, many with over 150 beds, and small homes are being bought by larger companies who then build extensions. The proposed emphasis on voluntary homes puts great pressure on the voluntary sector which does not generally have expertise in planning and running this kind of service. It is also important to note that it is not in the interest of existing home owners to have more homes opened in any district – profit margins are governed by occupancy levels, a high demand, short supply market makes their business much more secure.

Longer-term, planners will be facing a more fragmented service as the Government's plans for self-governing hospitals and more private community care services mature. It will be very difficult to draw up plans when the private providers can come and go at will. Serious doubts are being expressed, for example that other NHS reforms emphasise the division between the acute sector and community care, with little recognition that pressures on the acute sector are partly caused by poor community provision.

Achieving high standards of care

Caring for People aimed to provide inbuilt guarantees of high standards of care in both the public and private sectors. Emphasis on quality of services and quality of life for people in continuing care must feature in the contents of the plan for community care. The legislation and detailed policy guidance make it clear that plans for quality assurance and systems for safeguarding service standards, through stronger monitoring units, are to be established together with complaints procedures.

At a national level, there will be no specific Minister for Community Care, as suggested by Sir Roy Griffiths. The Social Services Inspectorate (SSI) have been given wider powers, the Audit Commission has extended its remit into monitoring health care, and health professionals have won a concession from the Minister of Health that a 'clinical standards advisory group' will be set up. This goes some way towards meeting the demand for an independent health care inspectorate – could it be extended to cover all patients, not just NHS contracted beds?

The White Paper proposed a system which was essentially designed to meet fiscal policy goals. There are, therefore, inherent tensions between the concept of 'value for money' and the high standards of care which are also called for. The wide variation in the way that value judgements are made by officers who register and inspect residential and nursing homes, suggests that national standards and guidelines for monitoring standards of care across all services will need to be introduced in the near future. Following the Wagner Committee's report, '*Residential Care: a Positive Choice*', there is already a government-sponsored development programme, aimed at testing and promoting ways of improving quality of life for people in residential homes. Will this bridge the gap between the standards expected in residential and nursing home registration and inspection criteria?

The training of registration and inspecting officers concentrates on the outcomes of care, dignity, privacy, choice, independence, rights and personal fulfilment, as well as the highest professional medical and nursing care for patients. The SSI publication *Homes are For Living In* (DoH 1989b), designed to monitor standards in residential homes, is also based on this approach. Everyone is entitled to basic human rights and sensitive personal care, let us hope that these new approaches to high standards of care will apply throughout the public and independent sectors.

We can learn from experience in other countries and anticipate the danger that pressures to produce more specific standards can have negative results, for example, if specifications become rigid and too prescriptive, as has happened in the United States. Each home must be measured against its own aims and objectives for care, within accepted guidelines, concentrating on whether it meets the standards which residents, as well as inspectors and managers, find acceptable. The new contracts for care, to be drawn up by social services seeking provision from a range of care providers, can hasten the moves towards high quality in those homes wishing to receive 'sponsored' residents.

Evidence to the House of Commons Health Select Committee by the Nursing Homes Associations indicated their concerns about the way that contracts may specify standards which are higher than those demanded for registration, particularly as the contracts are from Local Authorities who do not necessarily have knowledge and experience about nursing home provision. The contracts drawn up jointly between health and social services in Cheshire are an example of a contract which aims to improve standards of care. The London Borough of Sutton has conducted a care audit of homes and awarded 'hearts' to each. Homes must achieve one heart to be included on the list for contract in 1993/94, but will need to achieve standards which earn two hearts in the second year.

Registration and inspecting officers have developed considerable expertise, and could usefully have contributed to the discussions about service agreements between health, social services and private or voluntary organisations to ensure they are in tune. However, very few have been involved in this process and it seems possible that there will be considerable conflicts of interest between contract managers, placement officers and inspectors unless a dialogue is opened during the early stages of implementation.

Disagreements about standards have surfaced very strongly in some places in relation to proposals for dual registration of homes. Dually registered homes can provide a service in which individual user needs and preferences come first, and the public regulatory system has to be flexible to meet individual needs. It has proved successful in a few districts where political and managerial difficulties in registration and inspection have been overcome. The joint procedures and agreements developed by registration officers in health and social services, for example, in Cornwall, Worcester, Newcastle-on-Tyne and others, illustrate ways that a common system can be implemented, providing useful models for a standard approach across residential and nursing home care.

Monitoring standards

The Social Services Inspectorate issued guidance in 1991 to Local Authorities for the new 'at arms length' inspection units. _Inspecting for Quality_ has become the handbook for these new units, which inspect both independent and public residential care provision. Thus Local Authority homes and private or voluntary homes are now required to meet the same standards. Curiously, the present arrangements for the inspection of nursing homes by teams of Health Authority Inspectors is to continue, with all its inherent conflicts of interest heightened by the new relationship with the Local Authority.

At present, the legal basis of standards derives from the regulations under the Registered Homes Act (1984), which require home owners to provide 'adequate' standards across more than 20 items, from staffing to plumbing. Interpretation of these regulations are contained in guidelines produced by Health Authorities and Social Services Departments, and are based on The National Associations of Health Authority Handbook (NAHA 1985) and _Home Life_ (DHSS 1984) respectively. The reason for the changes in _Caring for People_ has become known as the 'level playing fields' argument: that, since Local Authority homes and geriatric wards are not registered, dual standards exist, to the disadvantage of the independent providers of care who must meet higher standards.

There can be no doubt about the severe impact of this change on Local Authority homes, especially when coupled with the financial disincentive for residents to choose a Local Authority home (which negates the 'level playing field' for Local Authorities in future). It has speeded up the sale of older Local Authority establishments which do not meet the physical standards, and which need large capital investment to bring them up to guidelines developed for the independent sector homes. It has also encouraged the transfer of the management of other homes to the voluntary sector, because many Local Authorities have had difficulty complying with staffing requirements and other high revenue costs. But the changes do not apply to NHS continuing care wards in geriatric, psychiatric or mental handicap hospitals, or to unregistered community units providing NHS services. The Registered Homes Amendment Act has brought small homes with less than four beds within the scope of registration, but the 'lighter touch' of Local Authority regulation means that these establishments may not be regularly monitored to ensure adequate standards. There are fears that although these homes may provide a cheaper alternative form of residential care, because fire regulations and other minimum standards are not required to be met, they may be used inappropriately for people who need more specialist services than can be offered in this setting.

The interface between health and social services, and between the public and private sectors may well become more tense as there are potential pitfalls ahead. The permutations are many, for example, what will happen if a Health Authority continues to register a home from which the Local Authority has withdrawn its contract on the grounds of poor quality of care? Conversely, there may be problems if Health Authority inspectors are unhappy with standards in nursing homes with which Local Authorities persist in maintaining contracts for services? Some parts of the country will have many more homes than others, will people needing residential care have to move far away from family and friends to find care at a price their Local Authority is willing to pay? Inspectors are already encountering resistance to improving standards in Local Authority homes, often because resources are simply not available, but there is a more startling anomaly. Inspectors cannot prosecute a Local Authority which fails to provide adequate care, however, this has become a regular method of achieving quick improvements in private and voluntary homes.

The impact of legal action against providers under the NHS and Community Care Act is severe. Provisions carried forward from the 1948 National Assistance Act include the mandatory clause that a contract shall not be placed with an establishment against which there has been a successful prosecution. Some Local Authorities are including the issuing of a notice of intent to prosecute in this prohibition. Thus the issue of an enforcement notice or successful prosecution for some minor, but persistent, failure could cause the closure of a home. This was not the intention of the registered homes legislation, and cuts across normal concepts of justice, leaving Health Authorities in a very difficult position. They must not ignore criminal breaches of the law, such as breaking of conditions of registration or failure to provide staffing in accordance with staffing notices, as this would be collusion with illegal acts, but taking action may result in closure from loss of contract – a far more drastic result than the fine imposed by a magistrates court!

Government guidance to Local Authorities in *Community Care in the Next Decade and Beyond* and *Inspecting for Quality* (SSI 1991) requires the publication of reports of inspections of residential care homes in the public and private sectors, but not those of Health Authority inspections of nursing homes. Service Commissioners in many areas are using published inspection reports as a basis for checking existing standards. Few Health Authorities publish reports, although there is no prohibition on this, leaving nursing homes themselves to make the reports available if they wish to bid for a contract.

The assessment of standards in residential and nursing homes is at present both haphazard and secretive. Public authorities often allow homes to continue to be registered which do not provide acceptable standards of care. This may be because inspectors prefer to assist home owners in reaching adequate standards, or because it is difficult to find sufficient evidence of poor care to bring legal action to close a home with which they are dissatisfied. The public have generally little information about which homes are considered good or bad. If consumers or users are to make real choices between staying at home or moving into residential care, the whole system will have to be opened up to public scrutiny. Potential users will need more than glossy brochures advertising public and private services, important though these undoubtedly are. Agreed standard measures have not been developed, and the debate about accreditation is as yet inconclusive.

The private sector argument for self-monitoring is not likely to find favour with users or the general public concerned about standards, although work is at present being undertaken by NAHAT in association with the Registered Nursing Home Association to produce a quality assurance accreditation system for continuing care. A monitoring system developed at Guy's Hospital (King's Fund 1988 "Achievable Standards of Care for the Elderly Patient" Project Paper 72), and adapted by Lewisham and Southwark Health Authority, provides a good example of standardised, objective assessment of quality. The methodology includes measures of input, process and outcome. This is the approach which could well provide the foundation for the national 'Quality Commission' proposed by the Labour Party (1989), with a user-orientated monitoring system for community care across all health and social service provision.

The registration and inspection officers working in DHAs and social services have often found it difficult to cope with their role at the interface between the public and the private sector. The new proposals will be welcomed because they raise the profile of inspection and recognise the importance of the work. Extra resources will be necessary if officers are to manage their expanded role, and training is needed to ease the adjustment from managers to monitors of care. As DHAs are merged into larger health purchasing consortia, nursing home inspection teams are being merged into larger units. Joint units with Local Authorities have been slow to develop, and reasons for this were researched for the Department of Health in 1992 (Brooke Ross 1992). Uncertainty about the future of county councils and changing boundaries add to the problem of planning joint working at all levels of community care. Inspection of homes is often the last thing to be resolved in local discussions, indicating a continuing under-valuing of this important function. Scandals of appalling bad practice continue to emerge from competent inspection and through whistle blowing to the media. The mixed economy of health and social care in the community cannot be left to grow unchecked.

Conclusion

The chapter has shown that, although there are many good proposals in community care legislation there are also many reasons for public concern. Attitudes to community care reflect the values that society holds for people who are disadvantaged by age, ill-health or disability. Many of the criticisms in this chapter have referred to care of elderly people because inadequate protection is offered to these vulnerable people under the NHS and Community Care Bill. The proposals for the transfer of people from Victorian psychiatric hospitals to the community most closely reflect Sir Roy Griffiths's proposals and deserve wider support, but even here inadequate levels of public funding and provision are already subject to much public criticism, particularly in relation to increasing numbers of homeless people with mental health problems, many of whom sleep rough in our cities each night.

Many criticisms are, not surprisingly, similar to those made about the NHS reforms. Each section of the National Health Services and Community Care Act 1990 reflects the Government's stated commitment to 'consumer' focused care, but each proposes a system in which professionals become gatekeepers to cash-limited services, rather than an alternative which opens opportunities for user choices. The Government's measures to limit public spending, while, at the same time, encouraging the expansion of publicly funded private services contain many contradictions, and make planning and budgeting increasingly difficult for Health and Local Authorities. Sadly, in the decade which promises *Health for All by the Year 2000* (WHO 1987) these reforms will widen the gap between people with private incomes and those dependent on state benefits.

It is vital that health and social services managers plan and provide services to meet the real needs and wishes of service users and carers. Many of the people requiring community care will need advocates to assist them in making their voices heard. The voluntary sector has fulfilled this role in the past, but is now to become a major provider of services. Far from clarifying 'who does what', the community care reforms leave voluntary pressure groups, care managers and inspectors of services with conflicting roles.

The relationships between the public and private sectors will undergo a fundamental change. Although closer cooperation and collaboration is demanded,this chapter has shown that there are many areas of potential conflict between health and social services. Everyone will need to work closely in a spirit of goodwill so that service users and carers can gain access to the ideal of 'seamless packages' of community care, which are designed to ensure that each individual receives sensitive,caring treatment, regardless of the status of the provider.

References

Audit Commission for Local Authorities in England & Wales (1986) *Making a Reality of Community Care* HMSO, London

Brooke Ross, R (1992) *Report of Joint Working in Inspection by Health and Local Authorities* Centre for Inner City Studies, College Hill Press, London

DHSS (1984) *Home Life: A Code of Practice for Residential Care* DHSS Working Party. Centre for Policy on Ageing

DHSS (1987) *Promoting Better Health* Cmnd 249, HMSO, London

DHSS (1989a) *Caring for People* Secretaries of State for Health, Social Security, Wales and Scotland, Nov, Cmnd 849, HMSO, London

DHSS (1989b) *Working for Patients* Secretaries of State for Health, Social Security, Wales and Scotland, Cmnd 555, HMSO, London

DoH (1989a) *Discharge of Patients from Hospital* HC(89)5 para A2, HMSO, London

DoH (1989b) *Homes are for Living In* Social Services Inspectorate, HMSO, London

Gatehouse, G (1990) NAHAT Conference Presentation

Griffiths, Sir Roy (1988) *Community Care – An Agenda for Action* HMSO, London

Hansard (1990) NHS and Community Care Bill, Second reading. 13 Hansard 169(70), London

HMSO (1984) *Registered Homes Act* HMSO, London

HMSO (1986) *Disabled Persons Act* HMSO, London

HMSO (1989a) *Local Government and Housing Act 1989* HMSO, London

HMSO (1989b) *Education Act 1989* HMSO, London

HMSO (1990) *NHS and Community Care Act* HMSO, London

House of Commons Health Committee (1993) *Community Care: Funding from April 1993* Third Report, HMSO, London

House of Commons Social Services Committee (1990) *Community Care: Funding for Local Authorities 3rd Report, Cmnd HC277, HMSO, London*

King's Fund (1988) *Achievable Standards of Care for the Elderly Patient* Project Paper 72.

Laing, W and Buisson (1989) Laing's Review of Private Healthcare

NAHA (1985) *Registration and Inspection of Private Nursing Homes: Handbook for Health Authorities* NAHA, Birmingham

Social Services Inspectorate (1991) *Inspecting for Quality* HMSO, London

Wager (1988) *Residential Care: A Positive Choice* Report of Independent Review of Residential Care, National Institute of Social Work, HMSO, London

WHO (1987) *Health for All by the Year 2000* World Health Organisation, Geneva

13 Working for patients . . . a public health perspective

Bernard Crump and Rod Griffiths

Introduction

The changes envisaged in the government's plans for the NHS, outlined in *Working for Patients* (DHSS 1989a) and the clutch of working papers that were published in its wake (DHSS 1989b, 1990), followed hard on the heels of guidance to District Health Authorities concerning their public health responsibilities. This guidance originated in the report of the committee of inquiry into the future development of the public health function which was published in 1988 (DHSS 1988a). The committee, which had been set up following two major episodes of communicable disease, both of which had resulted in public enquiries, was chaired by the Chief Medical Officer, Sir Donald Acheson. The committee adopted a definition of public health – the science and art of preventing disease, prolonging life and promoting health through the organised efforts of society – which was sufficiently broad to avoid their being confined to making comment on the management of infectious disease.

The combination of this broad definition of public health and the opportunity to rethink the pattern of health services that *Working for Patients* appeared to give seemed exciting at the time. Subsequent events proved once again that the NHS is a political system. Current patterns of care are anchored in place by perceptions of political risk as well as by some medical and other justifications. Large scale change, that seemed to be the Government's aim in enacting the reforms, was frustrated by the Government itself in a series of interpretations of the rules that allowed only GP fundholders to make significant changes. From this disappointing start how should the reforms now be viewed?

The public health responsibilities of Health Authorities, as expressed by the Acheson Committee and endorsed by the Government still make a good starting point to think about what may be possible and what has been missed so far. These responsibilities were:

1 to review regularly the health of the population for which they are responsible and to identify problems;

2 to define objectives and set targets to deal with the problems in the light of regional and national guidelines;

3 to relate decisions which they take about the investment of resources to their impact on the health problems and objectives so identified;

4 to evaluate progress towards their stated objectives;

5 to make arrangements for the surveillance, prevention, treatment and control of communicable disease;

6 to give advice to and seek cooperation with other agencies and organisations in their locality to promote health.

As these responsibilities are now enshrined in secondary legislation (DHSS 1988b) Health Authorities must decide how to carry them out within the new proposals.

The greatest major influences on life expectancy are genetic and environmental factors along with issues of lifestyle. The language of *Working for Patients* on the other hand suggests that it is underpinned by a model of health care in which hospitals play the major role. The lack of attention to primary care has since been rectified by the publication of the White Paper *Health of the Nation* (DoH 1992) that has re-emphasised the role of primary care and prevention.

This should have set the stage for radical change to be back on the agenda. However, a more pragmatic view would concede that, whatever their contribution to reduction in population mortality, secondary and tertiary services do reduce the burden of morbidity within the population they serve. Realistically, it is also the case that hospitals currently consume the large majority of the funds available to the NHS and this situation is unlikely to change in the near future. In line with Acheson's views, it is a public health duty of Health Authorities to ensure that all funds including those that are spent on hospital care are used as prudently as possible. Furthermore if hospital spending is not controlled and made to produce value for money as health gain then there will be precious little money left for anything else.

The proposals in *Working for Patients* seem to have got off to a bad start in terms of producing radical change but at the same time they are being blamed for whatever problems the service encounters. In a recession with heavy restraint on most sectors of public spending (unemployment benefit being the exception) the reforms are blamed when hospitals run out of money. It is not the purpose of this chapter to explain why some hospitals often run out of money at the end of the financial year but the reforms provide a new scapegoat. In some quarters the term 'crisis' has been used. In Chinese, the word for 'crisis' is represented by an ideogram which is made up of the ideograms for the words 'risks' and 'opportunity'. This image conveys an impression which seems very appropriate to the current state of the debate about

Working for Patients. What then are the opportunities and risks for the public health to be found in these proposals?

Opportunities

The most fundamental series of changes proposed in *Working for Patients* related to the introduction of a new relationship between those who will purchase services on behalf of a population and the providers, that is those responsible for managing hospital and community services. The clear intention was the introduction of a provider market. The task of purchasing falls to District Health Authorities, with an increasing number of GPs holding budgets with which to buy some services for patients on their list.

As a consequence of the establishment of NHS trusts, which has accelerated since the 1992 general election Health Authority non-executive and executive members are becoming less involved than they used to be in the day-to-day running of the hospitals and community services within the District. DHAs are more able to concentrate on assessing the needs of their population and seeking to purchase services aimed at improving health. Public health has become higher on the agenda of Health Authorities and, at least in theory, they are much better placed to carry out the first three of Acheson's five public health responsibilities for DHAs.

A further area for potential improvement relates to the way in which decisions are taken over the distribution of resources between priorities. Prior to the reforms a budget was set for each unit of management at the start of the financial year. Where activity targets were agreed, as part of the budgetary process, they were normally no more specific than to the level of speciality. Within these broad budgets and targets the providers determined the precise pattern of service that was offered. It was thus, in practice, not possible for the DHA to fulfil its responsibility to 'relate the decisions they take about the investment of resources to their impact on health problems . . .' since those decisions are being taken in a non-explicit fashion by clinicians. The clinician did not take into consideration the views of the district of residence when deciding to commit resources to treat a patient.

In the reformed NHS the purchaser places a contract with a provider for each service to be made available to a District's residents. The specification of contracts requires a number of steps:

- assessment of need in the population;

- identification of the service to respond to the need;

and where the appropriate response is the purchase of a health service:

- specification of the volume of service to be purchased;

- determination of quality standards to be applied;

- clarification of monitoring arrangements.

The processes involved in specifying and placing contracts are performed in a much more explicit fashion than has been the custom in the past. That is not to say that the views of clinicians will not be taken into account, but rather that they are incorporated into a systematic review of the relative contribution made by the spectrum of clinical activity to the health of the District's population.

Another criticism which has been made of the pre-reform methods of allocating scarce resources between priorities was the essentially incremental nature of the process, with an expectation that a particular service will retain 'its share' of resources from year to year. There was occasional talk of 'zero-based' budgeting but the nature of the relationship between districts and units was not conducive to radical reviews of service provision. The emergence of contracting could be seen as an opportunity to rethink the range of services to be provided, and to implement a discontinuous change in service development, though enthusiasm for radical shifts in the direction of purchasing has to be tempered with an understanding of the impact on providers and on patients 'in the system' with inevitable political ramifications. Whether Health Authorities seek or are allowed to pursue major change in their purchasing policies remains to be seen, though they were heavily constrained initially by the centrally imposed rules of the market that demanded a steady state.

One of the major public health problems to be faced by society is the extent to which access to health care is distributed inequitably within the population. The Black Report (DHSS 1980) and *The Health Divide* (Whitehead 1987) have demonstrated the extent of this inequality on a national basis, and the political sensitivity of the issue. On a more local level, Directors of Public Health have been preparing reports on the health of the population of their Districts, in line with the Acheson Committee's recommendation that such reports should be published on an annual basis. A common finding has been that, within Districts, access to services is not always equitable. This is particularly true where the District boundaries include inner-city areas or when the population is not socially homogeneous because of unemployment or ethnicity. A clue to the likelihood of such inequalities might be found from analysis for census variables in small areas, or by the use of aggregated scores such as Acorn, Jarman or Townsend (CACI, Jarman 1983, Townsend *et al.* 1988).

An example of such inequality was found in Central Birmingham when access to hip replacement was measured in each of the Local Authority wards in the District (Department of Community Medicine 1987). When the values were corrected for differences in age and sex between the wards, it was found that someone who lived in the most advantaged of the wards was seven times more likely to have an NHS hip replacement than a resident of the most deprived ward. No data was available to indicate the additional contribution of the private sector, which is likely to have meant that the NHS figures underestimate the real difference in access.

These differences are not uncommon, though the steepness of the gradient varies to some extent between diseases, and a few diseases such as breast cancer may show less treatment in poor areas. It is not difficult to speculate as to the reasons for these dramatic differences in access. More articulate patients, perhaps with more persuasive GPs, are more able to advocate for admission. There may be genuine differences in need between the residents of the wards, but it is difficult to justify the extent of the difference in access observed. Prior to the reforms the only method by which such inequality could be reduced was by pointing out to the clinicians involved that it existed, and reviewing procedures to ensure that there are no obvious causes.

Now it is possible for a district to place more than one contract for a particular service; indeed, for reasons of transportation it will be quite common for contracts to be placed with more than one provider for subsections of the population. It would be quite possible to redress inequality of access by, for example, placing two contracts for hip replacement, one for the more advantaged wards, the other for the more disadvantaged. The volume of service for which the contracts were placed could ensure equal access for the two groups or, more contentiously, could reverse the level of access.

A final major opportunity associated with the introduction of contracting lies in the ability to write measure of quality into the terms of the contract. Whilst many authorities have sought to improve the quality of services provided in their units since they were exhorted to do so by Sir Roy Griffiths in his report on health service management (NHS Management Inquiry Team 1983) progress was limited. In part, this can be explained by the perverse incentive which means that an improved quality of service, for example a new facility or reduced waiting list, attracted more referrals, often from neighbouring Districts, which conflicted with the need to stay within budget.

Under the new arrangements, providers who improve the quality of the service they offer should expect to attract more work, but also the funding to carry out the work. From the public health perspective, a major advance will be the opportunity for the purchasers not only to specify the volume and range of services which they wish to have made available for their residents, but also to be able to state standards of quality which they expect to see applied to the services concerned.

Broadly speaking, there are two categories of service quality which purchasers will have to consider. The first category, which is often dismissed by professionals as being superficial, concerns general features related to the experience of being in contact with the health care system. It includes issues such as waiting times, the environment of the hospital, patient information etc. These features are rather general and may not need to be specific to the particular service which a patient is to receive.

The second category is concerned with the quality of the outcome of the intervention which a patient undergoes. Clinicians have, in recent times, recognised interest in outcome to be a legitimate concern and the introduction of compulsory medical audit was met with broad agreement (Conference of Royal Colleges 1989). Increasingly purchasers of care wish to be able to assure themselves that the quality of service that they buy is adequate in both categories.

The introduction of the Patients Charter has led to the establishment of national or local standards for many of the more general issues. More specific quality standards of the second category are more usually particular to individual contracts. Whilst logically these more specific standards should relate to the outcomes of interventions in practice this may prove difficult. First, the time scale may mean that a contract is due for renewal before the relevant outcomes can be expected to have occurred. Second, if these standards are to be of value in monitoring the progress of contracts then the measures chosen should be wholly, or at least, largely, under the control of the provider. Thus, whilst the most relevant outcome to monitor in the case of a contract for acute myocardial infarction might be hospital fatality rate, this outcome is dependent on a range of factors, many of which are outside the provider's influence.

Whilst understanding of outcome measures improves, many authorities are trying to identify process measures that are closely associated with good or bad outcomes. These are sometimes called impact measures. Examples include delay in the use of thrombolytic therapy in patients with acute myocardial infarction, or annual numbers of similar procedures carried out by surgeons engaged in major oesophageal surgery.

Initial guidance suggested that purchasers should outline to providers the areas in which they wished to see standards set and monitored, with the providers setting the standards. Experience has shown the response to be patchy. Increasingly purchasers are becoming more pro-active in setting standards and some are beginning to experiment with ways of using the information that they receive after each admission to hospital as a trigger to generate their own data on impact, outcome and patient satisfaction.

The opportunity to write these quality standards into contracts, whilst it will involve a great deal of work to develop appropriate parameters, is a route by which the care of patients who need secondary and tertiary care can be improved.

Risks

If the previous section identified opportunities to benefit the health of the public that became available through the introduction of the proposals in *Working for Patients*, what are the attendant risks?

The basis of the economics of the market-place suggests that competition between providers will lead to increased efficiency of provision, through reduced costs, increased quality, or a combination of the two. Whilst the most radical, these are far from being the first attempts on behalf of Government to raise efficiency in the NHS. The financial stringencies of the last decade have led to reduced numbers of beds in most hospitals, but patient throughput has increased. Clinicians have been saying for a decade that the scope for further reduction in length of stay is slight, yet they have continued to occur (DHSS 1988c). It is not surprising that some managers and politicians are sceptical about some of the advice they receive from clinicians. There are obviously risks if civil servants, who have never treated a patient, ignore the advice of doctors; there are also risks if doctors exaggerate the danger of the new proposals.

The extent to which costs will reduce, and benefits increase, as the reforms bed down remains to be seen. One area in which the NHS could claim to be efficient, despite the popular folklore to the contrary, was in the cost of administration. There can be little doubt that the increased complexity of the new arrangements, with the need for Districts to place and monitor contracts and consult with GPs and for providers to cost and market their services and bill purchasers for the care they provide, brings with it increased administrative costs. Perhaps the biggest risk of the NHS reforms is that any savings from increased efficiency will be more than exceeded by the unavoidable costs of introducing the proposed systems.

A second risk relates to the extent to which the introduction of the new reforms has diverted the attention of Health Authorities and their senior officers away from other areas of priority. In the previous section, it was suggested that the arrangements might afford opportunities for DHAs to improve the way that they fulfil the first three of the five public health responsibilities outlined for them by Acheson. These benefits could be negated if the effort needed to make the most of the opportunities is so great that other work, perhaps less easily understood in the context of contracting for health care, suffers as a result. It is much more difficult to draw up contracts for services for people with learning disability than for hernia repairs. To some extent this risk was realised with the two year delay in introducing the community care elements of the Health and Community Care legislation (which came into effect at the time of writing).

Hard on the heels of the NHS reforms came the Government's plans for a national strategy for health *Health of the Nation* (DoH 1992). This document, which has been widely welcomed in public health circles, recognises that many of the major health problems facing us can only be tackled through collaboration with other agencies, so called 'healthy alliances'. This type of collaborative work needs skills, resource and time for it to bring benefits. These gains do not appear as shorter waiting lists or more patients treated and may not fit comfortably with the culture of a 'performance through contracts' NHS, particularly if their most accustomed practitioners are now engaged in contract monitoring and performance.

Two further areas of concern relate to the issue of commercial sensitivity. At present, a considerable amount of the data which can be used to build a picture of the health of a population is extracted from information provided by hospitals and community services. Private hospitals do not provide data of their activity; a fact that has meant that, particularly when considering elective surgery, and particularly in the South East, the information we have on hospitalisation is seriously deficient. It is conceivable that providers will not wish to provide this information in future, either because they do not wish for their competitors to have access to data on their activity, or because they wish to avoid the costs of data collection, encoding etc. Arguably, this source of data will be of even greater importance for the assessment of health in the future, and it is essential that it is not lost. Especially if their contribution to health care is to increase, the same data should be made available by independent providers.

A similar concern relates to the dissemination of the findings of research. In industry, if research leads to a new development, or a more successful approach to a problem, then the company will seek to exploit the commercial advantage afforded, and will not usually make widely known the details of the improvement. Until now, medical developments have been handled in a much more open fashion, with doctors publishing the details of new procedures and the results of their research; indeed, the importance of a good record of publications to professional advancement has provided an incentive to publish whilst no obvious disincentives have been in place. The competitive environment might lead to a less open approach, at least as far as the technical details of new procedures are concerned. We can take some comfort, however, from the situation of the USA where competition has not led to secrecy concerning medical developments; indeed, to some extent, a reputation built on research and publications may itself afford a competitive advantage.

Experience to date

It would be nice to think that a simple prescription could be written which would allow public health medicine to take advantage of the opportunities in the new arrangements whilst avoiding the pitfalls. In reality it is much too early to speculate as to the net effects of *Working for Patients*. Many of the opportunities for improving the health of the public depend on making the most of the contracting process but they also depend upon the process being allowed to operate in an unfettered way.

A series of new or improved methodologies will be needed if the chain of events from identification of need to the placement of a good contract with a satisfactory supplier is to be completed successfully.

The task is daunting, particularly when the need to consult with GPs and develop appropriate quality standards for the whole range of services made available to a population is considered. The best course of action for Authorities committed to fulfilling their public health responsibilities would appear to be to concentrate their efforts for change on a manageable number of health problems which they judge to be of most importance to the health of their population. For each of these topics a 'health plan' can be developed which will cover a limited period. The plan should start with an assessment of need based on local epidemiology and demography. This should be followed by a statement of the Health Authority's aims for reducing the impact of this health problem in the local population during the time covered by the plan. The publication of the White Paper *Health of the Nation* endorsed this selective process by setting out targets for health gain in five key areas. They were selected because they were important threats to health, or causes of mortality, and because there was clear evidence that something could be done about each of the conditions selected. Health Authorities were free to select additional local priorities if they felt that there was a strong local case but the same principles for selection should apply.

RHAs have the duty to ensure that DHAs have plans that should move their outcomes towards the *Health of the Nation* targets. Plans such as these will be the blueprints from which individual contracts will be designed and specified. Similar principles should underpin all plans but most authorities will focus their efforts for change in a few areas which will include the *Health of the Nation* targets. This clear emphasis on health gain should prevent too much attention even in aggressive providers from being directed towards the less acceptable face of marketing, namely the process of increasing demand until it reaches the level of supply.

Monitoring contracts

One area in which the Department of Public Health will expect to be involved is in monitoring the contracting process. Whilst monitoring contract compliance is not the same as monitoring the public's health, there is considerable overlap in the data and methodology to be employed. The Department of Health will shortly announce new views about the role of Regional Health Authorities. It already seems clear that they expect there to continue to be an intermediate tier between the Department and Districts but it will employ far fewer people and take a much more hands-off approach.

Health care delivery can be analysed as inputs, process and outcome. Each presents a different opportunity for monitoring. In terms of inputs, there will be a clear need to know, at any point in time, the volume of service available and not yet consumed for each contract. Clearly, for elective procedures, it will also be essential to know of patients who are waiting for admission. This raises the question as to where the responsibility for the waiting list lies; with the purchaser, or with the provider. Clearly, if the contract is of cost and volume type, the purchaser must accept responsibility for those patients who are referred after the contract volume has been expended. Up to this point, the responsibility for managing the waiting list is best placed with the provider. In the case of block contracts, it could be argued that the onus should rest with the provider, at least until an agreed number of patients have been treated under the terms of the contract. As the majority of provider units become Trusts and the focus of RHAs shifts towards purchasers we should see the beginnings of waiting lists based on District populations and a consequent shift of responsibility towards purchasers. They would then be expected to change the type of contract to one that ensured reduction of the waiting list.

It is also possible to monitor the extent to which the population seeks care outside the contracts which the DHA has placed, so-called extra contractual referrals. The new financial arrangements ensure that systems will be in place which will facilitate the monitoring of inputs. In terms of process, broadly, it is necessary to monitor the extent to which the provider is complying with the terms of the District charter, and with those specific quality issues which have been included within the contract. The systems currently in place to provide Korner and other statistics are of limited value here. Traditional process measures – length of stay, throughput etc – may be easy to collate, but new *ad hoc* systems will be needed to address the majority of the measures. In essence everything worthwhile about the reforms, in terms of seeking improved quality, has the downside that a new way of monitoring it will have to be implemented.

Turning to outcomes, the situation is similar. Measures of outcome of health care can be considered to fall into three categories – mortality, morbidity and satisfaction. We are quite good at measuring mortality, though if the death occurs in someone who has been discharged from hospital, we seldom relate the two events, though work is in progress in some regions to begin to develop indicators of this sort (West Midlands Regional Health Authority 1992). Measuring morbidity, whilst not easy, is eminently possible. Again, current systems do not allow easily a health care intervention to be linked to a subsequent measure of morbidity; if the morbidity measure is carried out by the person responsible for the original intervention, it may be subject to bias and could be wasteful of resources. 'Review' clinics are largely a thing of the past. If anyone else makes the measurement, for example the GP, the person responsible for the original care is unlikely to hear about it and if they do, they may not believe the results.

The softest of the three types of measure, that of satisfaction, is widely mistrusted by professionals but certain to increase in importance. A point worth making is that for hospital and community services, the term 'consumer' must be considered to include the GP as well as the patient. It can be argued that GPs are best placed to monitor the distant outcomes of hospital interventions and that, albeit not in a very explicit fashion, their referral decisions reflect the experience of similar patients who they have managed in the past, and should not be lightly regarded.

It is widely agreed that outcome measure should be our aim. Indeed, these measures are not only important for monitoring contracts, but many are also the measures of public health needed to assess need. Outcome measures will only be of real value if they are linked to each other, and to other health and life events. The proposal in Annex 13 of Working paper 11, on the information requirements of District Health Authorities (DoH 1990) that DHAs should consider the development of a health events register which will build a cradle to grave picture of the health of their residents, was greeted with enthusiasm by those in the field of public health, tinged with some cynicism as to the ability of the health service to deliver such a system in a workable form. In the mean time, most Districts should expend their energies in the identification of process measures in which the association with a beneficial outcome has been demonstrated, or is self-evident.

Conclusion

The approach to *Working for Patients* which is outlined here, one which is pro-active and population based, is a major change for many of those who were used to the more traditional concerns of District Health Authorities. Whether the non-executive directors of DHAs will be well equipped to function in this environment remains to be seen. What is clear is that they will need advice from professionals who are familiar with the range of skills that will be needed to support this work, including epidemiology, principles of health economics and the ability to evaluate the impact of health care interventions. Thankfully, there is no sense in which the purchasers of health care can be seen to be in competition with one another and it is to be hoped the Districts will feel able to share the expertise which they develop and their solutions to problems which they all will have to face; indeed, arguments have been developed for reducing the number of purchasing authorities considerably. It seems likely that the political emphasis on structural change will continue. Opponents blame NHS failures on the structure and process of the reforms and propose new changes, whether they be mergers of new forms of organisation or new roles. In fact this is a distraction from the fact that health care is provided by dedicated professionals and public health is best safeguarded by good epidemiology, good management and a bias towards primary care and prevention. None of these things come about through organisational change. The great advantage of the reforms could be that they make decisions more explicit and they thus give those who run the NHS the chance to see clearly what they should be doing and make changes where they are most needed.

References

CACI Market Analysis Division, 59–62 High Holborn, London, WC1V 6DX

Conference of Royal Colleges and their facilities in the UK (1989) *Building on the White Paper: Some Suggestions and Safeguards* Proposals for discussion from the Conference of Colleges. Circulated by the Royal College of Physicians, 17 July 1989

Department of Community Medicine (1987) *A Picture of Health* CBHA, Birmingham

DoH (1990) *Working for Patients* Report of the Project 34 Working Group

DoH (1992) *The Health of the Nation* Cmd 1986, HMSO, London

DHSS (1980) *Inequalities in Health* Report of research working group, HMSO, London

DHSS (1988a) *Public Health in England* Cmd 289, HMSO, London

DHSS (1988b) HC88 (64)

DHSS (1988c) *Comparing Health Authorities, Health Service Indicators, 1983–86*HMSO, London

DHSS (1989a) *Working for Patients* Cmd 555, HMSO, London

DHSS (1989b) *Working for Patients* Working Papers 1–11, HMSO, London

Jarman, B (1983) 'Identification of underprivileged areas' *British Medical Journal* **286,** 1705–9

NHS Management Inquiry Team (1983) NHS management inquiry (Published under cover of a letter from Roy Griffiths to the Secretary of State for Social Services) DHSS, London

Townsend, P *et al.* (1988) *Health and Deprivation: Inequality and the North* Routledge, London

West Midlands Regional Health Authority (1992) *Quality and Outcomes Indicators: a First Report* WMRHA

Whitehead, M (1987) *The Health Divide: Inequalities in Health in the 1980s* Health Education Council, London

14 How does it really feel?
John Dennis

Introduction

Working for patients was essentially concerned with changes in structure, management and culture. The first and only function of health care management is to provide as much high-quality care, both disease prevention and cure, as possible in the interests of the consumer with the level of resources which can be generated. Management arrangements must therefore be judged on the degree to which they facilitate effective working practices and provide leadership and support to all areas of direct patient care. Each successive restructuring must ultimately be judged by the improved health status of the population served, given at least parity of resources or the ability to generate resources. It must take into account consumer expectation in the widest sense as well as the enormous advances in medicine and health care.

Aims and objectives

Working for Patients provided some clear aims and objectives. These included:

1 That there should be better care and greater choice for the patient achieved by:

- emphasising the outcome of care as the measure of quality and effectiveness of the service using such techniques as medical audit;

- distinguishing the buying and providing roles so that authorities could offer choice of secondary care venue seeking the best buy rather than looking towards the local service;

- involving general practitioners in the buying process through developing priorities in conjunction with the Local Health Authority with the option of practice budgets.

2 That there should be greater cost-effectiveness on the part of the provider achieved by:

- money following the patient;

- developing the buying and providing roles;

- introducing capital charging so that Authorities should take a realistic attitude to estate and equipment assets;

- introducing the notion of Trust status as a means of further instilling private sector motivation into the public sector.

3 That providers should be rewarded for good performance achieved by:

- money following the patient (this in fact means the patient's data);

- a clear responsibility for providing to meet needs;

- further delegation of power and responsibility to the local level.

How then does the service have to operate if the Government's aims are to be achieved, since these are, in theory at least, arguably a reasonable basis for good quality care in major parts of the service, aims which have at least to some extent become clearer with a greater degree of commitment to the *Health of the Nation* in particular.

A coherent structure

The first point to make is that *Working for Patients* essentially addressed secondary care services and seeks to deliver better quality care and choice in hospital care. It does not address primary care, health promotion or disease prevention in detail and therefore only partially addresses the continuum of care although as stated above, *Health of the Nation* makes some attempts to address this as indeed does the Tomlinson report for Inner London, *Making London Better.*

Even taken with the more recent White Paper *Caring for People* the problem of a cohesive, complementary and properly orientated service needs to be given a great deal of further thought. The latter paper focusses on such vital issues as proper assessment and collaboration between agencies to plan delivery together at the individual (case management) and total service levels and seeks to introduce the notion of the mixed economy into residential and nursing home delivery just as in the hospitals system. The near future will clarify this.

We must therefore encompass the Government's aims in a local structure in which 'money follows the person'. Health care investment should therefore:

- seek to establish the highest achievable health state for the individual by advising on healthy lifestyle choices;

- prevent disease, eg through vaccination and immunisation programmes;

- provide help and support in the home as independence diminishes;

- provide supported accommodation as dependence increases;

- provide hospitalisation during episodes of acute illness.

In such a structure:

- The District Health Authority/Local Purchasing Authority must be free to set policies and priorities in and between client group services, reflecting central guidance but responding to local epidemiology and demography.

- The District's resources must be invested in the community. The management structure in the community must be capable of assembling realistic and usable individual care plans and aggregating these into a business plan for a geographical locality (the patch) which responds to primary and secondary care needs within the District's policy and priority guidance. Concepts of the patch or locality will I believe change as the influence of the GP on primary and community care increases by direct purchase or otherwise.

- The organisation must be capable of developing the language and technology to describe health needs in expected outcome, quality and quantity terms. As a result, the purchasing authority will be able to carry out its buying role through a contract with local primary care managers, with secondary/hospital providers either within or outside the District reflecting best buy and patient preference. Total packages of care from either an integrated Trust or by the joint arrangements of two separate Trusts will become commonplace. There would seem to be an enormous overlap between the interests of the District Health Authority and the Family Health Services Authority and this will continue to be overcome with emerging arrangements.

As this concept is developed, there will be the opportunity for a mini-RAWP type approach to neighbourhoods/patches within the catchments. Areas of special need/deprivation will have the greatest opportunity in conjunction with the general practitioners in the patch to take most from the agreements-contracts negotiated by the Health Authority. Indeed, as the organisation closest to the customer, not only the general practitioner but also the patch manager will be expected to contribute to the agreement reflecting local needs – needs both in terms of prevention, community care and secondary/hospital care.

The mixed economy

Early agreements have largely been characterised by a formalising of what formerly took place. This has been no bad thing because the current level of information is generally insufficient to enable more radical decisions to be made in most areas. There will be the opportunity to change this more radically over a period of time. Furthermore, one should not underestimate the high political charge which will associate with the potential change which a genuine market would encourage. Additionally, whilst the United Kingdom has very different geographical characteristics to those of the United States, nevertheless the 'deserts of care', which are characteristic in certain parts of the USA, cannot be allowed, nor can the enormous cost of billing and processing by providers and payers estimated by some as 1 per cent of the American GNP and indeed at $44.3 billion similar to the total cost of NHS and associated care in the UK. A more realistic billing system will avoid the commitment of this kind of resource. General practitioners have generally not felt the same responsibility to the local provider and when large consortia of fund holders are coming together greater changes can be expected.

Management capability

Underlying these arrangements in all aspects of the service is the ability to describe good quality, quantity and fair price in a manageable and unerstandable form. The NHS must therefore reach a lead position in the use of technology. It must also be faced that investment in the management capacity required to provide and measure a good service to the consumer does not come cheaply. The kind of organisation that performs as we would wish to see it in the future cannot afford to glory in low management overheads. Management overheads of 5 per cent would not keep major commercial and industrial companies to the fore and nor will it sustain a high quality/efficient health service. A realistic level might be in the order of 10–14 per cent. Though this will produce a lean service focussed on priority issues, it is unlikely to make up for the crude service reduction arising from diversion of 6–10 per cent of consumer service into management. It is unlikely that there will be a significant addition in resources for the NHS in the short term. There will be an increase in the sums required for management and its supporting infrastructure. This resource can only be made available from areas of patient funding initially and, before any advantages from competition can develop, there is the potential for loss of care. Longer term, there is the opportunity for real advantage and increased levels of quality and quantity. It may not be a comfort to know that the highest priorities are now being met when one's own position on the hospital waiting list is worsening. I believe that the area of greatest significance is the role of clinicians in the management structure. In provider Trusts where greatest success is being achieved in terms of changes to meet changed needs, consumer choice and the economic situation, the clinician is very much part of management and a leader in it. There is a great deal wrong with the culture of the service when this is questioned. It casts doubt on the various professional bodies that it is not automatically seen as such.

An information 'visionary' had a dream. It went something like the following:

The general hospital in question was fortunate to receive sufficient funding to implement HISS by selecting a modern Integrated Hospital Information System (IHIS).

Seventy year-old pensioner, Harry Jones, was brought to the accident service at the hospital on Sunday night. The junior doctor who saw him was assisted in her diagnosis and initial care plan by an 'expert system' which formed part of the A&E computer. The personal details given by Harry's wife had also been entered into the computer, which had retrieved Harry's case notes which were stored on optical disc, revealing his history. Combined with the doctor's original assessment this information was sufficient to suggest that Harry be admitted immediately to a medical ward. The computer revealed that no bed was currently available on the appropriate ward, but that one should be available by mid-morning, if Dr Jenning's ward round confirmed Mr Smith's progress to be satisfactory. The bed was therefore 'reserved' on the computer and Mr Jones was placed on another ward till morning. In the meantime, requisite drugs and blood tests were requested, using the 'order communications' module of the software, and the computer had already generated bar-coded labels for the specimen bottles and a bar-code wriststrap for Mr Jones. When the drugs were dispensed the following day, the bar-code labels were again used, and the stock control module of the system automatically recorded their issue and checked for possible re-order. In the laboratories, the specimen bottles received were checked against the overnight order received and the results were returned to the ward again via the 'order communications' module. Simultaneously, the main database was recording the tests and drugs ordered in Mr Jones' medical history, which was available to his doctors and nurses for the planning of care. The information about Mr Jones – particularly the assessment of his nursing dependency – when combined with the similar information about the other patients on her ward enabled the sister to determine whether she had sufficient nurses of an appropriate skill mix to manage her current patients, enabling her to release a nurse to a neighbouring ward.

At the end of his stay, the information collected about Mr Jones' care, as a by-product of its ordering and delivery, was sufficient to provide his general practitioner with a comprehensive picture of his time in hospital. This comprehensive picture of the services received by Mr Jones, along with his diagnosis, also provided the hospital doctors and managers with the information to assess the quality and cost of his care against preset profiles and standards for the care and cost of patients with conditions of that type. Indeed, the budget of the clinical department, which conducted his treatment, was reduced in line with the prices set for the various items of service he received, and these 'costs' were credited to the budgets of the support departments providing them.

A summarised file of Mr Jones' care was also transmitted over the wide area network to the District Health Authority he lived in (determined automatically by the computer from his postcode). The Information Support System there, contained a comprehensive population health register, and was able to verify that Mr Jones was a genuine resident of that area. As the population health register was also shared by the local community health service, general practitioners, and Local Authority Social Service, Harry Jones' keyworker in Social Services was able to alert meals-on-wheels to resume their service, and arrange for a follow-up visit by a health visitor for elderly people. The general practitioner was also able to review the discharge summary on-line, and request open-access physiotherapy from a local hospital. The District paid the hospital for the treatment by credit transfer, and had another patient flow statistic in its planning database. Apart from the labels, paper was never used.

It is unfortunately likely that this will remain a dream for the immediate future at least. Moreover the 'vision' did not take account of the advantages to be gained from the fact that Mr Jones had an NHS number which allowed a quick check to update on care which he had recently received whilst visiting relatives in other parts of the country during the last year. (Countries which were members of the EEC could not contribute information as yet to take into account details of an accident sustained on a recent holiday on the Continent.)

The rationing process

But, is there a function for waiting lists in the future? It might be argued that the traditional rationing system is a function of time and the historical background of the local service so that a GP might have said 'I'll put you on the waiting list but your problem isn't that serious and the hospital hasn't a very big department in your specialty anyway. So you're likely to wait a long time'.

Today there is a specified level of service expressed in a District's or fundholder's contract and reflecting the judgement of general practitioners. Therefore, a general practitioner would be saying, 'You have a condition which we don't regard as dangerous or seriously impairing your quality of life which we have not given a priority in the contract for hospital services agreed with the District Health Authority or which we have negotiated as a fund holder. We cannot offer you a service'. This puts pressure on Health Districts to consider the existing contract as well as alternative sources of provision. This dialogue at the general practitioner level will not only highlight the need for GP–DHA communication on priorities but might provide an environment where more minor priorities/procedures are carried out more appropriately by general practitioners. This contact is required even with the increase in spend of the GP fundholders. There must be a coming together of purchasers if the service is going to develop beyond that of a day-to-day or at least year-to-year forecast to meet immediate needs.

If this sounds callous, then it shouldn't. At the moment, we let people remain on waiting lists with no real prospect of (or in some cases need for) treatment. They are the people who are or feel disadvantaged. By having a clear and explicit understanding of priorities we can ensure that the right people do get prompt attention. Without sizeable increases in resources or the results of greater competition, the outcome of the White Paper is likely to be that a different, but 'right' group of people do not get a service.

It will certainly change the role of the general practitioner. In particular, the general practitioner recently graduating from the GP rotation programme will wish to have the opportunity to undertake a number of the procedures which may be currently referred to the specialist. Where a meaningful dialogue between consultant staff and general practitioners has taken place regarding referral and aftercare, the guidance and advice on both sides has led to changes in referral and discharge patterns. The financial incentive will be only one aspect of the change in the way certain needs are met. General practitioners will wish to take advantage of any leasing opportunities of minor operating theatres and certain diagnostic facilities. This will lead to a greater partnership between the GP and not only the community services but also aspects of secondary care.

Working for the consumer

How can we give the future service the consumer bias which its might be expected to have in a market system? There are a number of vital initiatives, mostly recognised in the working papers on contracting. As well as measuring clinical quality through medical audit, we must also measure the patient's satisfaction. What did the patient think of the doctors, the nurses, the catering, the pre-admission arrangements and the receptionist's smile? This information must be used by providers seeking to win/keep market share and the buyers seeking to award value for money contracts. It will be interesting to see how the introduction of the league tables influence consumer choice. A new market could be envisaged for publications associated with '*The Good Health Guide*'!

Service providers will, therefore, develop a marketing capability in order to survive. They will need to understand and exploit the media as would any large-scale organisation in an increasingly competitive market-place. The efforts that the American hospital often makes to improve this market share through improving the concept that the local population has of it are as competitive as in any other sector. Updates on performance will appear regularly in local media.

There will need to be a 'style' to care delivery. Ideally, it will be demonstrably consumer centred – the notion of the hospital patient as a guest might be a useful challenge. This notion would need to be constantly in the forefront of every member of staff's mind since all staff will appear in the shop window at some time and some staff at all times. The staff are the main salesmen in any organisation. Different parts of the organisation will need to be more supportive of other parts, particularly if the Trust provides services of an integrated nature, every member of staff is a salesman for the corporate entity. There will be a need to break down professional jealousy and to develop a "corporate" identity.

Market policy will also need to be precise:

- What range of services must I offer to go to the market with a strong portfolio?

- What services are my strengths and the mainstay to my sales strategies?

- What services are my weaknesses and do I want to remedy them?

- What are my competitors' strengths and weaknesses?

- What services do I want to reassess in order to strengthen my overall market share?

- Where can I make profits to invest in the indirect areas of the operation which I need to improve:
  - patient amenities;
  - management/IT development?

- What is the image which I want the public to have of the organisation?

- Is this image fully understood and supported by staff within the organisation?

The buyer/provider relationship

The operational principles Working Paper 'divides' purchasing authorities from provider units. The principle of clear responsibility and account-ability in the NHS does need to be further developed in line with the general management principles introduced as a direct result of the Griffiths Inquiry. However, it will become even more apparent that the clarity of purpose and responsibility does not imply in real terms a loss of working together between the buyer and provider generally.

Providers must be free to take decisions as to how best to deliver care to the patient but the modes of delivery must clearly reflect the expectation of the principal buyers. The contract/agreement is the formal point of contact, but successful companies prosper with the less formal approach in addition. It is not a matter of agreeing a contract and then making contact at the end of the contract period or when it fails to be met. Better systems of monitoring contracts both by the purchasers and providers will develop and the value of the face-to-face discussion will be more appreciated. Dialogue must be on a regular basis. Contracts will be varied with agreement throughout the period based on changes to need and pressure, information availability and good sense. The maxim 'both sides have to make a profit' will become paramount, particularly as there will not be full market conditions, even in large conurbations. I question whether GP fundholders will make possible complete patient choice. The close relationships between buyer and provider is best illustrated by two outstandingly successful organisations Marks and Spencer and Peugeot Talbot. In the performance of these companies preferred providers are generally small in number. Information and technology is essentially shared. Contracts are for a sufficiently long period to benefit investment plans and other factors of both sides. The buyers and providers in the NHS who will be successful in implementing enormous change in a limited period will be those who can work together and be determined to keep it simple.

When considering aspects of pricing and cost there is the need to highlight the issue of investment. The provider will not want to undertake innovation into new lines which could deflect from current activity, effect prices for 'the current lines' and thus market share, without support from the main purchasers. The Trust is therefore dependent on the purchasing authority for its future 'business plan' just as the purchasing authority is dependent on the Trusts for provision of new services.

Buyers cannot, as the Working Papers state, be reliant on providers for product specification. This will be drawn up jointly using the buyer's knowledge of what is wanted and options put forward by the provider as to how this might be supplied. The end service to the client must be 'bespoke' not 'off the peg'. Major purchases for human resources will not be purchased from a seed catalogue or even from a holiday brochure, although it will become more obvious that there are a number of similarities between purchasing health care and a vacation – the information technology element rather than the outcome.

The purchaser/purchaser relationship

This has already changed perhaps more rapidly with mergers and other arrangements than was at first realised. Some of the more obvious areas of overlap have not been grasped. It is inevitable that these changes will have to be made. Large purchasers however can result in loss of appreciation of local opportunities through the inability to study micro problems and plan and prioritise together effectively within these areas. Again the worst effects of this can be minimised by close purchaser provider working including planning. Historical patterns of provision need to be challenged.

Purchasers will work more closely with other purchasers. There will be a greater exchange of expertise, a willingness to exercise joint accreditation and perhaps specialisation between allied purchasers. The Regional Health Authority has an opportunity to encourage this but will need to develop a philosophy or culture under which it can develop this – one in which purchasers clearly can see the benefits and one in which Regions are able to monitor the key performance areas of improving the health of the population which is the ultimate and only aim of purchasing bodies. This will become an even greater challenge in the event that Regions under whatever guise become associated with the health status and lifestyles of larger populations. This will lessen the charge that Regions in some instances are too interested in detailed Provider issues.

The greatest change in the purchaser relationship must be that between the main purchasing authority and the GP whether fundholders or otherwise. I do not believe that the main purchasing body can perform without close working with the general practitioners and in particular the fundholder. The multi-funds of GPs may help to obviate this, but I believe that it will be well into the decade before even the multi-funds are in a position to develop a strategic approach to purchasing rather than to concentrate on present needs and the strengths and weakness of current providers. There will be an 'umbrella' group for forward planning. A body at present difficult to envisage beyond the purchasing authority, will be expected to monitor GP purchasing contracts within the overall strategy. The concept that the work currently undertaken by the DHA/FHSA/GPs including fundholders and the Local Authority with particular reference to the Social Services can continue without the greatest cooperation is nonsense. There is perhaps the need for a 'holding company' for these activities. Perhaps this 'holding company' could include 'people representatives' through a CHC nomination.

The provider/provider relationship

The concept of setting up independent trusts within the NHS does not, initially at least, encourage the closest of relationships between these independent providers. The future economic situation makes it probable that there will be a continued squeeze on resources. I am far from sure that a clear evaluation was undertaken prior to *Working for Patients* that this would result in the decrease in the cost of health care and if so by how much under the revised arrangements. Financial pressures will dictate changes which are enforceable at least in part through a contracting system. As this bites further into the resources available, it will become necessary for providers to work more closely with providers. Many people working within the NHS would be surprised at the degree of cooperation which exists between competing providers in industry and commerce. Mergers in the commercial and industrial world are common place both friendly and otherwise. This will develop into the 1990s and interest will quicken as public and private mergers become commercial options. Incidentally, I believe that providers will be even more vigilant as to the opportunities for private patient care development on site and the need for improved cash flow. There will be a greater realisation that some of the key personnel are working for a competitor (this in terms of both private and NHS competitors where 'cooperation' has not been established). There will be a major surge in joint ventures although this will remain somewhat marginal in terms of total capital and revenue spend. "Spare capacity" will offer both a challenge and an opportunity.

The health service as a market – the market and the planning role

The rational planning policy would be to secure the maximum local accessibility (subject to acceptable quality and cost) for all services.

In a free market system an ideal market might be defined as 'a provider looking for a lot of buyers and a buyer looking for a lot of providers'. Health care is not a free market system given the responsibility of the purchaser to secure care for its home population.

Working Paper 2 (paragraph 2.10) associates 'block contracts' with core services on a three-year, rolling basis. Both 'block' and 'cost and volume' contracts afford the opportunity to specify quality, range, quantity, performance and cost issues.

The purchaser should view the widest possible range of services as core services where it can secure a 'monopoly purchaser' position and thus have services provided when, where, and how it wants them. In this way it can retain its planning function – ie it can influence not only the quality and quantity of existing services but influence providers to develop new services. This does not mean that it cannot take advantage of market forces to improve the quantity and quality of service negotiated, but change will at least initially be very much at the margins.

It should use the appropriate contract mechanism for each core service, eg block contracts where the emphasis is on a service which needs a certain capacity to respond to demand (accident services, obstetric services etc), cost and volume contracts when the requirement is for a given level of service for work where there is a significant elective element. It is quite possible to predict emergency levels within a specialty and to include them in a cost and volume contract.

The opportunities for those working for the service

The NHS is already beginning to look very different to those employed within it as the pace of change intensifies. The British culture does not welcome change as readily as certain other nationalities. The change is being introduced at a time when a demand for many specialties is increasing. Certain of the professions see their influence decreasing (will their contribution be included in the agreement/contract in the face of competition). The level of funding can change dramatically with the loss of a contract with its implications on staff, training and estate. It is inevitable that the ratio of 'non-established' or 'temporary' non-core staff will increase to overcome the less predictable future. Staff will be expected to be more flexible in the manner in which they contribute to the organisation. There is an enormous future for the organisation and its staff which becomes a truly 24 hour operation maximising staff and other resources for the full 24 hours in line with patient preference and clinical and economic good sense.

The medical profession

The emphasis on involving the medical profession in management is being given added thrust on the back of *Working for Patients*. The clinical directorates will continue to become more the norm in the provider units. There is the opportunity to influence to a greater extent the individual consultant contracts at operational level. There will be a need for a major input of training to overcome in certain instances the absence of formal management experience and formal training. Unless this is undertaken, there will be an unnecessarily high turnover of directors, full advantage will not be taken of improved technology, there will not be bringing together of the various professional interests and, perhaps the worst scenario, a divide between the directors and other medical staff and staff in the directorate generally.

It will be the clinical director who will need to have more involvement in the contract process – both in terms of discussion with the buyer as well as acting as the bridge with clinicians in any one directorate, to deliver the quality and quantity of care within the appropriate time and within agreed costs. There must be some concern that the high level of managerial tasks placed on the clinical director will persuade all but the most managerially ambitious to decide to concentrate on direct clinical activities. The 'in turn' process will not be effective in appointing clinical directors.

The medical profession have the opportunity to lead the quality aspects of the agreement/contract through the work of the audit groups. Failure to realise the importance of this will lead to a degree of frustration as zealous contract managers push the frontiers of quality forward.

Other direct patient care staff – staff generally

The nursing profession have not taken full advantage of the managerial changes and this undoubtedly has been a loss to patient care. Providers who do not maintain a clear role for a senior nurse in the hierarchy run the risk of not maximising the skills and standards of this key workforce. Furthermore, nurse management has a major part to play in the clinical directorates and this can include the leadership of them. Nurse management must become more involved with general management. Likewise, the various therapy services are becoming more aware of the need to obtain their own particular 'market share' within the organisation – where this approach is taken and the service delivered, the contribution will be recognised. I believe that there will be strengthening of the emphasis on the development of therapy with associated staff in the community or non-hospital setting. The therapist will continue to have a major influence on certain key factors such as length of stay. The therapist particularly when able to work within an integrated Trust can greatly influence the need for admission as well as length of stays.

The more entrepreneurial will, I think, grasp the opportunities to set up business units or agencies. In addition to the various therapy services, this will include the estates, financial and personnel and training functions. The likelihood is that certain of these will be subject to management buyouts in a later phase. This lead has occurred at Regional level, not always successfully.

Staff, I believe, will be encouraged by the increasing opportunities for local negotiations over salaries and associated conditions. Providers will need to develop greater skills in this area.

Health care personnel are a very diverse group with different expectations and horizons. However, there is an enormous degree of cooperation in spite of what are often difficult employment conditions. Initial confusion and resentment must be overcome by good communications, a realistic and sensible timetable and training where necessary. The attempt to create more responsibility and authority at local level can lead to greater purpose. Initial change should concentrate on what is really beneficial and really necessary to gain these benefits. I believe that members of staff do want to share in the success of a department or unit. If given clear objectives and feedback on success, I believe that all will perform willingly in the changing environment, most especially if it can be seen that the patient is benefiting. The importance of staff incentives is paramount, as indeed is that for the organisation as a whole. This does not necessarily imply a financial incentive.

The chief executive

It is the chief executive who is most responsible for the change whilst at the same time maintaining responsibility for the current service being delivered.

Working through to the implementation of *Working for Patients* and beyond, there will always be periods of elation and frustration. The value of key staff will be appreciated, particularly when their talents are recognised by another employer. The chief executive will need to manage through far greater uncertainties than previously.

There will be a continuing change in relationship between the chief executive and other senior managers. There will be a changed emphasis on certain skills – the greater importance of the commercial activities, including marketing – negotiating for health care contracts – the opportunities for the greater use of information technology in decision taking, and local negotiations with staff including senior medical staff—in other words personal business development.

The relationship between the chief executive and the clinicians will remain as ever of major significance and even more significant will be that between the executives and non-executive directors. I believe that the role of non-executives has already changed enormously from the former one of a 'member'. The successful boards will be those which can harness the various skills of all board members, executives and non-executives.

However, for the provider the business remains the delivery of health care, health promotion and disease prevention – and the chief executive's activities in the past and in the future must reflect this.

Conclusion

So what will it look like for the patient as we move through the 1990s? Perhaps it would be more sensible to consider the second half of the decade rather than the immediate. Such a monumental change in a short period leads to confusion. Professional and political interests, unfortunately, often magnify this. Once again, it will appear very different to different people in different places. Where the implementation has been carried forward in conjunction with the various agencies, ensuring a very close relationship between essentially the buyers, providers, the general practitioners and statutory and other bodies, including voluntary organisations, the transition can best benefit the customer. Where it is implemented without this cooperation and without the full involvement of staff, services will not be maintained certainly in terms of quality. Urgent discussion between buyers and providers will be required to rectify problems. There is the opportunity for the patient to receive a more personal service. A degree of choice must emerge. There is a clearer incentive through high levels of work being rewarded with resources to match this level. This can only be achieved however, if the purchaser is able to recognise the need for incentives for better performance by the provider.

I believe that the momentum being built around quality and outcome will develop to the benefit of patients and staff. However, the question must be asked as to the extent that the political factor will allow market forces to come into play and or the consumer to be able to make a high degree of choice. The degree of risk has shifted from the purchaser to the provider. The skills of providers in handling this as well as ensuring that the purchaser does not off-load all its responsibilities is paramount.

There remains a great future for the National Health Service. It is strongly supported by the public. The new arrangements and systems will enable a better case to be made for an increase in healthcare's expenditure as a percentage of GNP, even if not to the levels of the USA of approximately 13 per cent in the 1990s. It must retain all that is good from the past, together with the best of the opportunities which changes offer. It must develop a culture which seeks out change rather than waiting for (and perhaps resenting) the change which is thrust upon it. As we learn and experience more of the benefits of *Working for Patients*, we can move forward into new areas and opportunities. Some doubts remain to be clarified – this includes the fundamental one of the clarification (and a degree of honesty is required) as to what the Government is committed to do and to state clearly what it intends not to do. The ability of general practitioners to act as the 'insurance agents' for health care gives some cause for concern. The NHS has I believe suffered from the lack of a balance between short-term and long-term planning. I am not certain that we have necessarily achieved the mechanism for this. The 1990s clearly have the opportunity to refocus community and secondary care balance and to ensure that care and disease prevention is provided in "the Right Place".

Index